COCAINE

Studies in Industry and Society

Philip B. Scranton, Series Editor

Published with the assistance of the
Hagley Museum and Library

Recent titles in the series:

COCAINE

From Medical Marvel to Modern Menace
in the United States, 1884–1920

Joseph F. Spillane

The Johns Hopkins University Press

BALTIMORE AND LONDON

© 2000 The Johns Hopkins University Press
All rights reserved. Published 2000
Printed in the United States of America on acid-free paper

2   4   6   8   9   7   5   3   1

The Johns Hopkins University Press
2715 North Charles Street
Baltimore, Maryland 21218-4363
www.press.jhu.edu

Library of Congress Cataloging-in-Publication Data
will be found at the end of this book.
A catalog record for this book is available from the British Library.

ISBN 0-8018-6230-2

CONTENTS

ILLUSTRATIONS

ACKNOWLEDGMENTS

The years spent researching and writing this book would not have been possible without the assistance of many people: students, colleagues, advisors, friends, and family. For all those who have offered support and encouragement, I am most grateful. Special thanks to the faculty and graduate students of Carnegie Mellon University, where this work began life as a dissertation. My advisor, Steven Schlossman, never failed to challenge me to think about the historian's work in thoughtful and creative ways, a challenge that I hope is at least partially realized here. For his support of this project, I am greatly indebted. Many thanks also to Mary Lindemann as a member of my dissertation committee for numerous critical readings. My fellow graduate students taught me a great deal during our time together, especially Timothy Haggerty and Jennifer Trost. Very special thanks go to Jared Day, graduate school colleague and good friend. My appreciation goes also to the faculty and students of the Center for Studies in Criminology and Law and the Department of History at the University of Florida.

Much of the research for this book was made possible through the generous support of the RAND Corporation Drug Policy Research Center, with funding from the Alfred P. Sloan Foundation. Particular thanks to Peter Reuter, former codirector of the center, for his interest in initiating this project and for many useful comments and suggestions. Thanks as well to another former codirector, Jonathan Caulkins, for ongoing support of the project and enthusiasm for its goals. Other important financial assistance was provided by a Drug Information Association dissertation summary award and by the University of Florida.

The willingness of scholars whose interests crossed mine to share their knowledge and insight never failed to amaze me. In large and small ways, their assistance has made this a better book. Three persons in particular helped me through sources in the fields of medicine and pharmacy: Jonathan Erlen of the University of Pittsburgh, Gregory Higby of the American Institute for the History of Pharmacy, and John Swann of the Food and Drug Administration. I also wish to thank the following persons for their help: Caroline Acker, Jim Baumohl, John Burnham, Robert Byck, David Courtwright, J. Worth Estes, Paul Gootenberg, Mark Haller, Jill Jonnes, Mara Keire, John McWilliams, David Musto, Ethan Nadelmann, Glenn Sonnedecker, and James Harvey Young.

The task of locating and identifying source material took me to many libraries and archives, where the librarians and staff offered their expertise and interest. In particular, I wish to acknowledge persons at the following: the Bentley Historical Library at the University of Michigan, the Chicago Historical Society, the Chicago Public Library, the Burton Historical Collection at the Detroit Public Library, the Falk Library of the Health Sciences at the University of Pittsburgh, Hunt Library of Carnegie Mellon University, the National Archives, the History of Medicine Division of the National Library of Medicine, the Lloyd Library and Museum, the Regenstein Library of the University of Chicago, special collections at the University of Illinois–Chicago Circle Campus, and the Western Historical Manuscript Collection at the University of Missouri–St. Louis.

Series editor Philip Scranton offered enormously valuable support and advice as well as a critical reading of the manuscript. Where I followed his suggestions, the book is the better for it. Senior editor Bob Brugger of The Johns Hopkins University Press proved patient and encouraging and helped to make this project a finished reality.

Finally I would like to thank my family, without whom this book could not have been written. My wife's family provided encouragement, especially Barbara and George Stackfleth, historians both. Thanks and much love to my family for making this appear possible many years ago, especially my parents, Joseph and Judy Spillane. My love and thanks most of all to my wife, Jennifer Stackfleth Spillane, who sat side by side with me in more archives than she cares to recall and who saw to it that our daughter Margaret never took second place to a book manuscript. Above all, her support and encouragement of my work inspired its completion.

COCAINE

Introduction

At the end of the twentieth century, cocaine seems central to the American drug problem. After several decades at the margins, cocaine experienced a resurgence of popularity in the 1970s. Cocaine consumption grew to an estimated 300 metric tons in the next decade and has remained at comparable levels to the present day. Cocaine captured the popular imagination, first as the "jet-set" drug of the cultural elite and then as the "inner-city" drug of the socially marginal. In between, assertions of the dangers of cocaine helped justify a renewed and expanded war on drugs. Much has been made of the "newness" of the cocaine threat to public health and safety. Cocaine has been made to seem a drug without precedent, a drug whose long history has been lost.

The most recent cocaine experience is not America's first, however. A century ago, doctors introduced cocaine as one of the most important contributions of medical science to health and well-being. Over the course of three decades, cocaine grew from being a medical wonder drug to an important player in American drug culture. In the process, although it remained legally available in most states until after 1900, the drug's growing popularity sparked a movement to control its unregulated use and distribution. The resulting wave of state and local legislation culminated in the passage of the federal Harrison Narcotic Act in 1914 and the introduction of national drug prohibition. This critical transformation — from unregulated medical marvel to tightly controlled social menace — became the foundation for contemporary drug prohibition and is the primary subject of this work.

Policy discussions since the 1970s demonstrate only a dim awareness of this early history, and the paucity of historical context to the contemporary drug control debate might well be regarded as justification enough for an extended historical inquiry. Indeed, several recent commentaries have pointed to a need for historical experience to inform decision making.[1] With such encouragement, it is hard to resist the temptation to use the past as a primer on current drug policy, but there are potential pitfalls to such an approach. Perhaps the most serious of these is the creation of a kind of antihistory of cocaine, which relies on pharmacological consistency at the expense of social and historical context. The first generation of historical inquiry produced a good deal of this type of work, dedicated to little more than locating and cataloging historical instances of cocaine use — the early experimentation of Sigmund Freud, Arthur Conan Doyle's creation of a fictional cocaine-using detective, even the endorsement of a famous French coca wine (Vin Mariani) by Popes Leo XIII and Pius X — all intended to contrast the enthusiasm of past generations with the relentless disinterest and hostility of the prohibition regime.[2] Such an approach, almost antiquarian in its method, located cocaine in a variety of interesting places, from Coleman's Toothache Drops to Coca-Cola, but explained little about its uses, intended and actual audiences, or settings of sale. The first aim of this work, then, is to locate products and personalities associated with cocaine in their own historical time and place.

The importance of historical context helps explain why this work focuses on cocaine alone rather than on the whole range of substances subject to legal controls during this period, including opiates and alcohol.[3] The idea of "drugs" is both a social construction and a legal fiction, useful for regulatory purposes but hardly helpful for sorting out distinctive substances. This work deals with the preprohibition period, when the unique benefits, effects, and costs of cocaine formed the basis for drug-specific policy. Adding to the complexity of this story, many in the preprohibition era also distinguished the coca leaf, the source from which the alkaloid cocaine was extracted, from cocaine. These considerations emphasize the need to take "cocaine" seriously as an independent phenomenon and as a substance with a distinct history.

If the central theme in the history of cocaine is its transformation from medicine to menace, the theme of modernity is the constant that bridges the two eras. Two traditions in the existing historical and social scientific literature, broadly distinguished as constructionist and objectivist, provide a foundation upon which to build an analysis of these issues, but they too often seem at odds with one another, mutually disinterested at best. In dealing with cocaine as a modern drug, this work aims to combine the strengths of each approach.

The constructionist approach emphasizes how drugs might be understood as the product of social concerns and understandings that give substances an identity beyond mere pharmacology. An enormous variety of work has built upon this basic premise, from early studies showing the effects of setting on the drug experience, to more vigorous challenges to the concept of addiction itself.[4] The literature on the creation of social problems effectively demonstrates the extent to which persons' interpretations of social conditions shape their definitions of the problem. Much of the most important work in this area has examined the creation of legal prohibitions, starting with Joseph Gusfield's pioneering study of alcohol prohibition and including Marek Kohn's recent work on the birth of the British drug underground, in which he concludes that "the outlawing of drugs was the consequence not of their pharmacology, but of their association with social groups that were perceived as potentially dangerous."[5]

American responses to cocaine resemble the British experience. To critics, cocaine revealed the dark side of modernity; new and frightening patterns of popular cocaine use followed from the degeneracy and disorganization produced by industrial society. Even worse, the effects of cocaine were widely believed to reinforce, and even accelerate, the very social problems that produced the impulse toward drug use in the first place. The "story" of cocaine was told directly through visual representations in which cocaine was pictured as a serpent, a dragon, or a demon, seducing and torturing at the same time. The most potent of all of these images was that of the degraded users themselves, the so-called *cocaine fiends,* described by one observer as "a strange, uncanny tribe."[6] These images gave life to cocaine and animated the fears and anxieties of a modernizing society viewing a new drug culture.

Although the constructionist perspective most often deals with the process by which drugs became a social problem, this approach also helps to make sense of the enthusiasm for cocaine. Cocaine eventually came to represent the dark side of modern life even though its crystals once appeared to reflect the light of scientific progress and industrial achievement. For medical science, cocaine served as a powerful example of progress through modern laboratory experimentation. For the users of cocaine, the drug sustained the "modern" body — besieged by stresses, the brain and body could be restored by the invigorating properties of cocaine. Even in the subsequent underground drug scene, the cocaine experience seemed to elevate buyers and sellers to the top ranks of the modern world — a young user in Pittsburgh described the sensation of feeling "like Andrew Carnegie," and a dealer in Chicago fashioned himself "the Rockefeller of dope."[7]

The objectivist approach to examining drugs as a social problem, in contrast, treats drug selling and drug taking as objective phenomena that can be measured, counted, and classified with some precision. If cocaine was a construction, it was also a commodity, and recent studies from a number of disciplines on drug markets suggest a new objectivist framework within which historical change might be apprehended. One line of contemporary research employs a "market" approach that incorporates social and cultural context and the ways they change over time. The preface to a recent study of European drug markets describes illicit drugs "simply as commodities" that "shape and are shaped by demand and supply, exchange and consumption." Another line of contemporary research takes an ethnographic approach to the participants in drug markets, including work on upper-level drug dealers in California and more recent studies of street-level cocaine sellers in New York City. Historical research into other forms of illicit enterprise have also suggested ways in which drug markets might be apprehended. As Mark Haller observed, "in order to understand such activities . . . it is necessary to ask the same sorts of questions that would be asked concerning any other retail business activity."[8]

Examining cocaine as an object of manufacture and exchange is quite congenial to social history (and indeed, business history) because it takes seriously the ways in which individuals organized the cocaine trade. Understanding cocaine to be a manufactured commodity reveals a great deal about the timing of its popularity because the drug was among the very first substances to benefit from the newly expanding research, production, and distribution capacity of a rapidly modernizing pharmaceutical industry. With cocaine, drug companies sought to shape demand rather than simply respond to consumer interest. Later, the decline in popular cocaine use was aided by the willingness of many drug manufacturers to accept the demands of the emerging cocaine control effort to limit consumer access to the drug.

Images of cocaine in the popular press gave the drug one kind of life, but daily transactions between buyers and sellers also animated the drug experience. "Details" such as drug form, dosage, route of administration, price, and purity mattered to consumers quite as much as social labels and moral crusades. However flexible the constructions of cocaine, a customer entering a drugstore in search of coca-enhanced red wine would not have accepted a cocaine-enhanced suppository as a substitute. The most significant development in the retail cocaine trade before the Harrison Act — the creation of an underground market — reflected the neighborhoods and vice districts in which the business flourished.

This social-historical approach helps explain why, although this work is largely about the legal use and distribution of cocaine, it takes great care to avoid reliance on law or legislation as a historical marker of change. Although the critical transformation from modern drug to modern menace certainly owed something to political efforts at a national level, undertaken by prominent figures whose actions and motivations have been well documented and recorded, much of the relevant "action" took place on the street, in the daily interactions among sellers, users, families, doctors, police, and jailers. When a sixteen-year-old from Chicago's West Side visited a nearby drugstore in search of a cocaine powder for himself and some friends, the result depended less on the legality of the transaction than on the willingness of the druggist to complete the exchange. Specific actions in cases like this are, of course, harder to document, but this work proceeds from the notion that they are as important to the transformation of cocaine as is the passage of legislation.

One moves, perhaps inevitably, toward a reconsideration of legal prohibition itself. Critics and supporters of drug prohibition tend to date "modern" drug history from the passage of national antinarcotic legislation. Yet the history of the legal use of cocaine demonstrates how unimportant certain legal milestones actually were; statutes such as the Harrison Narcotic Act merely affirmed changes well under way before 1914. As a consequence, the later chapters of this work pose a series of questions intended to challenge traditional thinking about the impact and the legacy of drug prohibition.

First, to what extent did the legal prohibition of cocaine lead to the conditions now so commonly associated with the black market? As far back as the passage of the Harrison Act, it has been an article of faith among prohibition critics and supporters alike that drug laws created underground sales, low purity, uncertain quality, drug adulteration, and high prices. The restriction of legal supplies by formal control certainly reinforced all of these trends; more questionable is the implicit assumption that lawmakers imposed their will on a free and open drug market. The picture of the preprohibition drug market must take into account the informal rules that influenced the transactions between drug users and sellers. Self-regulation of legal distribution made equal consumer access impossible; social and cultural judgments about the appropriateness of certain kinds of exchange created a climate in which an underground market could actually precede restrictive legislation.

Second, did restrictive legislation stigmatize cocaine use and its users? Here too, critics of the prohibitionist regime effectively demonstrate the ways in which the law reinforced the demonization of the drug user, but they overstate the extent to which these negative images were absent in the earlier period. Ethan Nadelmann offered a summary of the critical view with respect to opiate addiction: "Many opiate addicts, perhaps most, managed to lead relatively normal lives and kept their addictions secret even from close friends and relatives. That they were able to do so was largely a function of the legal status of their drug use."[9] Yet by the end of the 1880s, strongly negative stereotypes already figured prominently in public discourse, exemplified by one description of cocaine users as "a very caricature of manhood."[10] The rapid acceptance of the "cocaine fiend" concept points to the need for closer examination of social attitudes in the preprohibition period.

Third, what was the relationship of drug control to other areas of social reform and state regulation? A purely legislative history risks devoting too much attention to the rhetoric of control. Public debates over the dangers of cocaine, although provocative and interesting, tell us a great deal about political agendas but relatively little about the process of building a regulatory apparatus. The passage of the first federal regulation to deal with cocaine in consumer products, the Pure Food and Drug Act of 1906, illustrates the need to consider the process carefully. Although the Act provided the Bureau of Chemistry with fairly weak police powers, Bureau Chief Harvey Wiley exploited relationships with professional organizations such as the American Medical Association, muckraking journalists, and the drug industry to achieve a much stronger state authority than the formal legislation implied. The existence of these public/private networks also makes it easier to determine in what sense legal controls "worked." This multiplicity of impulses explains why formal controls were so ineffective, did so little to improve the lot of cocaine users, and failed to reduce the cocaine trade dramatically. The different impulses behind reform allowed legislation to fail as drug control because it produced other satisfactory outcomes such as the establishment of broader legal authority over drug development and marketing.

The first cocaine experience in America did, finally, come to a conclusion of sorts. By the 1930s, cocaine had largely disappeared from the popular drug scene, moving to the farthest margins of a drug culture dominated by opiate use, not to return again for several decades. Did prohibition work? Were other factors, unrelated to formal policy, responsible for the decline? This work concludes with a reassessment of the impact of prohibition in light of this review of the preprohibition era. The story contains, above all, no clear "before" and "after" but a process of buying, selling, and understanding cocaine which continues to this day.

ONE

A Miracle of Modern Science

The Medical Use of Cocaine

On October 22, 1884, former President Ulysses S. Grant arrived at the office of Dr. John H. Douglas, one of the leading throat specialists in New York. Grant had begun experiencing severe throat pains that summer and sought out Douglas on the advice of noted Philadelphia physician J. Chalmers DaCosta. Douglas examined the general's throat and determined that Grant was suffering from incurable throat cancer. Douglas recognized that Grant's suffering would almost certainly increase as the disease progressed. To treat the pain, he turned to cocaine, a new drug that promised to provide considerable relief. Douglas treated Grant with topical applications of a cocaine solution throughout the course of his terminal illness.

That Douglas should have administered cocaine at all owed much to the remarkable coincidence of Grant's first visit in the fall of 1884. Less than a month earlier, the New York–based *Medical Record* published a letter from an American ophthalmologist in Vienna concerning the previously unknown anesthetic properties of cocaine. The *Medical Record* correspondent had observed a young Austrian physician, Carl Koller, announce the results of an experiment in which he had anesthetized the surface of an eye with a solution of cocaine. The medical elite of New York, including Douglas, immediately recognized the potential impact of Koller's work on surgical and general therapeutics.

Within weeks, surgeons across the United States adopted cocaine in ophthalmological operations. In the following months, the utility of cocaine as a local anesthetic encouraged its expansion into other areas of surgical practice, and its efficacy in surgical therapeutics prompted countless American physicians to experiment with applications in general medical practice. In less than a year, cocaine had become one of the most promising new therapeutic agents of the medical profession.

Cocaine, previously little known, now embodied the promise of modern medical science. The emerging scientific goal of grounding medicine in laboratory experimentation called for a new approach to drug development. Physicians increasingly urged that the physiological effects of drugs be thoroughly tested and evaluated in the laboratory. As one of the premier new products of laboratory research, cocaine heralded this exciting new age of drug therapeutics.

Physicians identified several of the effects of cocaine to exploit in medical practice: mood elevation, topical anesthesia, stimulation, and pain relief.[1] The apparent reliability of these effects encouraged a medical profession widely dissatisfied with existing drug therapies. Even when physicians recognized that cocaine had only a palliative, rather than a curative, effect, they appreciated the relief and satisfaction their patients (including former President Grant) expressed.

The medical use of cocaine was never indiscriminate or faddish. The months after Koller's dramatic announcement were full of excited and overenthusiastic praise for the new substance, but in practice, the many proposed applications for cocaine soon narrowed to several common uses: as an anesthetic; in the treatment of opiate addiction (and sometimes alcoholism); as a tonic that reinforced and stimulated both body and mind; and in the treatment of various sinus conditions (including colds and hay fever).

The medical literature reveals a significant range of therapeutic practice with regard to dosages, forms, and routes of administration of cocaine. In general, physicians handled cocaine quite conservatively, prescribing low dosages and short-term treatments. Lower-potency coca leaf preparations found great favor for their tonic and stimulant benefits. In some areas of medicine, however, the use of cocaine was less restrained. The treatment of opiate addiction and sinus ailments was notorious for encouraging the use of frequent and large doses of cocaine. This diversity of therapeutic use highlights the need to examine the early history of cocaine in the context of nineteenth-century drug development and medical practice.

The Coca Prelude

When Carl Koller conducted his investigations in 1884, he did not "discover" cocaine itself but rather its first important medical application. Chemists in Peru and Germany, roughly twenty-five years earlier, had isolated the alkaloid from coca leaves. Since the sixteenth century, European travelers to South America had observed the use of the coca leaf to increase stamina and reduce feelings of fatigue and hunger. European scientists who traveled to South America in the early nineteenth century reported the sustaining power of coca. In a typical account, a Swiss naturalist observed in 1835 that "moderate use of Coca is not merely innocuous, but that it may even be very conducive to health." He marveled at the Indians who chewed coca three times a day over the course of years and who "nevertheless enjoy perfect health."[2]

Centuries of occasional reports from South America resulted in little sustained effort to popularize coca. After the Civil War, however, a small group of physicians reexamined the therapeutic potential of coca. Doctors in the South and Midwest employed coca as a stimulant and published their findings in several regional medical journals. There is little evidence, however, that these coca enthusiasts convinced large numbers of physicians to employ coca in their practices. On the contrary, the advocates of coca remained on the margins of the medical establishment in the eastern United States, which gave little credit to their observations.

Cultural hostility toward the claims of Latin American coca users contributed to the skepticism. Although travelers to South America often left convinced of the properties of coca, those who read the accounts second hand remained unmoved. Coca advocate W. Golden Mortimer wondered that it "seems almost incredible" that a substance that so many had used for so long was ignored in the United States, considering that so many travelers had noted its properties. Unfortunately, Mortimer concluded, these "travelers' tales" were widely regarded as flights of fancy induced by a "rarefied atmosphere" and an "exalted desire to enhance the wonders of travel."[3] John Uri Lloyd, a well-known eclectic physician, remembered that before Koller's discoveries, "physicians using coca were made subjects of ridicule, as being incapable of judging a remedy's qualities . . . while the natives who employed it in their daily life, as well as the travelers who were impressed by what they had observed of its effects, were regarded as involved in ignorance, or imbued with superstitious imaginings."[4] Physicians regarded observations of "native" uses as a poor source of information for civilized medicine. One physician flatly declared to Mortimer that it would be foolish for a reputable physician in the United States to adopt coca because "the Indians are great liars." Still others wondered if coca might have different effects on Indians than on the more civilized constitutions of European and American users.[5]

Difficulties in obtaining coca compounded the skepticism about its efficacy and formed an obstacle to experimentation by its advocates. Coca leaves frequently spoiled and lost their active properties while being shipped to Europe or North America.[6] The transportation of coca leaves from the growing regions of Peru and Bolivia was still difficult enough in the 1870s that supplies were notoriously low, prices high, and quality very poor. Coca leaves on the United States market varied markedly in quality, with many inert leaves sold.

William Searle, a New York physician and one of the early advocates of coca, obtained his first specimen of the leaves from Peru in 1865, a 25-pound bale that "had, however, been six months on the way, had suffered from the curiosity of the custom-house, and had thus lost much of its virtue by evaporation of the volatile element." Searle proceeded to use what he had at hand, and "chewed up the majority of the bale without any other effect than a lessening of the appetite and some increase of physical endurance." Although Searle decided to press forward with his work on coca, this first experience left him "quite incredulous of the stories told of the effects of Coca." Searle wrote to physicians in Peru, who assured him that "fresh leaves were in fact quite different in appearance from those which he had used."[7]

Problems locating reliable coca supplies collided with the emerging consensus that new therapeutic agents should be tested thoroughly in the laboratory. Increasingly in the late nineteenth century, those who urged that medicine should be grounded in experimental science called for a new approach to drug use by physicians. This new model recommended that the physiological effects of drugs be carefully tested and measured. Uniformity in drug action would then assure uniformity in treatment and therapeutic effect. The new model of physiological laboratory research challenged older patterns of empiricism in medical practice, which had their origins in French medical philosophy in the early nineteenth century. Empiricists posited that the observations and experience of individual practitioners would develop therapeutic practice most effectively. In contrast, as John Harley Warner suggested, "advocates of this newer model believed the physician's identity should derive less from an interaction with patients and other practitioners, [and] more from an allegiance to science (defined especially as that of the research laboratory)."[8]

Along with this new devotion to the products of the laboratory came a commitment to so-called *physiological therapeutics*. Physiological therapeutics involved measuring precisely the effects of particular remedies on bodily functions. This included directly observable changes as well as modifications in specific physiological processes such as pulse rate, temperature, and composition of the urine. Understanding when and how changes in these physiological states might be manipulated could then guide treatment.

Many of the early coca reports were clearly not the kind destined to impress the skeptical. Physicians who demanded detailed information on the physiological observations more often found clinical observations offering little or no explanation for why coca did what it did. One doctor, writing in the *Louisville Medical News,* put his views directly: "to be brief, he got coca and got well."[9] More important, the poor quality of the coca supply affected the physiological research that *was* conducted. Because so much of the available supply of leaves was inert, researchers were unable to reproduce in the laboratory any of the effects its advocates claimed for coca. In the 1870s, G. F. Dowdeswell, an English physician, conducted well-publicized laboratory tests on the physiological action of coca. The results of his research suggest that Dowdeswell was using a preparation made from inert leaves. Unable to produce any physiological changes with coca, Dowdeswell concluded that coca had no value "either therapeutically or popularly" and that a "more decided effect" could be obtained from "tea, milk-and-water, and even plain water, hot, tepid, and cold."[10] Being compared unfavorably with water had obvious negative implications for the therapeutic use of coca leaf preparations!

Defenders of empiricism (and coca) attacked skeptics by deriding their commitment to physiological research. Searle argued forcefully that it was "ridiculous" to deny the utility of coca merely because laboratory experimentation "cannot yet give the how or why." To do so, Searle concluded, was akin to denying "the growth of a blade of grass because we were ignorant of the processes of its development."[11] John Uri Lloyd pleaded "for tolerance of thought and action toward men *who know that which they know* by reason of *personal experience,* and the art of empirical observation."[12]

No person articulated the early antipathy to coca better than Edward R. Squibb, a member of both the American Medical Association and the American Pharmaceutical Association and head of an important pharmaceutical house. Squibb had long criticized the quality of the national drug supply, characterizing many of the drug products arriving in the United States as "low grade" and calling for greater regulation and inspection.[13]

Squibb pursued his own coca research but found the poor quality of coca on the American market frustrating, complaining that his search for good coca was almost invariably unsuccessful. Instead, "the best that could be done . . . was to accept occasional parcels, the best of which were of very inferior quality, and therefore unfit for medicinal uses, and these at very high prices." Squibb observed that "it is pretty safe to say that nineteen-twentieths of the coca seen in the United States market within the past two years must be almost inert and valueless, yet all is sold and used, and its reputation as a therapeutic agent is pretty well kept up."

Squibb compared the "florid stories of travelers," which endorsed the use of coca, with Dowdeswell's research, which suggested that coca was a nearly inert substance. He acknowledged that there were "fewer observers" on Dowdeswell's side but concluded that his laboratory research was thorough, extended, and accurate. On the other side, the "more or less enthusiastic travelers" had not used "modern methods of precision." After several years of frustration and disappointment with coca, Squibb determined to abandon its use altogether. He declared that it would no longer be sold through his pharmaceutical firm, and he regretted only that he had not discontinued it earlier.[14]

Medical Research and Cocaine

Ironically, only months after the publication of Squibb's final denunciation of coca, physicians in New York received the first word of Carl Koller's experiments with cocaine in Vienna. A sensational development in the history of anesthesia, Koller's work opened the floodgates on research into the physiological effects of cocaine.[15] The same philosophy that rejected the unproven claims of coca users embraced cocaine as a true product of modern research and scientific experimentation.

William Oliver Moore was among the first physicians in America to learn of Koller's work. At a meeting of the Medical Society of the County of New York, Moore read a paper entitled "The Physiological and Therapeutical Effects of the Coca-Leaf and Its Alkaloid." Moore reported his observations of the physiological effects of cocaine upon several animals and then detailed the results of self-experimentation with the drug. Moore noted that small injections of cocaine numbed his skin, dilated his pupils, increased his pulse, and raised his temperature slightly. The speed with which physicians had come to learn of Koller's work and to expand upon it, Moore concluded, "was a marvel" that "went to show that it was one of those substances that had 'come to stay.' "[16]

The surgeon general's *Index Catalogue* lists many similar studies, with titles such as "The Physiological Action of Cocaine on the Frog," "Cocaine and Its Influence on Bodily Heat," "A Study of the Action of Cocaine on Circulation," and several dozen others.[17] Laboratory research of this kind was just beginning to exert an influence over medical practice; the cocaine experience served as a useful example for those who sought to justify such experimentation.

Investigation of the utility of cocaine in surgical therapeutics led to interest in the potential scope of its applications in general medical practice. Charles Castle of the Cincinnati Eye and Ear Clinic noted that the excitement and information generated by surgical studies, including his own work, opened up cocaine to general therapeutic experimentation and use. Pioneer laryngologist Francke Bosworth first observed the vasoconstricting effects of cocaine when he used it as an anesthetic in nasal surgery. Based on these observations, Bosworth suggested the applicability of cocaine in treating nasal polyps, head colds, hay fever, and swollen sinuses.[18]

As the packing and shipping of coca leaves improved, the available supply grew rapidly in 1885, encouraging a great deal more research on the physiological action of cocaine. The results of these investigations suggested additional applications in general medicine. J. M. DaCosta of Philadelphia read of the effects of cocaine on the eye, and like many other physicians, he was inspired to conduct research "with a view to ascertaining whether it might be of use to the physician as well as to the ophthalmologist." DaCosta's work focused on the hypodermic administration of cocaine. Observing the effects of cocaine on the body, DaCosta found that the pulse became "fuller and stronger" and that the body temperature increased slightly. Applying these findings to therapeutics, he concluded, "The effects on the pulse and temperature recorded in these observations, suggest its application in many a condition of collapse, of weak heart, or heart failure; and its employ in low fevers, too, as a cardiac stimulant is a self-evident proposition."[19]

In addition to this kind of original research, physicians sought to test older therapeutic claims for coca. Claims ridiculed as superstition only a short time before now became the subject of intensive study. In the process, applications derived from centuries-old traditions were transformed into miracles of modern medical science. Roberts Bartholow, one of the leading advocates of the new physiological research, wrote in 1891, "No remedy in modern times — probably in any age of the world — has become so famous in so short a time as cocaine, and no remedy has so soon been subjected to the tests of physiological experiment and clinical observation."[20] Even allowing for some partisan exaggeration, cocaine clearly embodied the hopes of some in the medical profession for a new age in medical practice.

Numerous medical accounts observed that the most striking feature of cocaine in practice proved to be its contrast to existing remedies. By 1884, physicians employed relatively few drugs on a regular basis, and many of these were under attack by those who doubted their efficacy. Even a popular drug such as morphine had been attacked as overused and dangerous. Where skepticism was the order of the day, the arrival of cocaine was most welcome. Medical journals heralded a positive new era of drug development which would replace the "rubbish" of existing pharmaceutical therapy.[21] Francke Bosworth exclaimed that "we finally have at least one [drug] which never fails us" and that, in a famous phrase, "were it a question with me whether I should abandon cocaine or the whole of our Pharmacopoeia besides, I would unhesitatingly prefer to retain the cocaine."[22] Even Squibb, who had so roundly condemned coca only months earlier, marveled at the potential of the new alkaloid. Rarely, in his experience, had a "novelty" been so readily taken up for medical trial. Even more rare, Squibb admitted, was to find such a drug "so very definite and so very important in its results, and the future utility of which is so quickly and so easily established."[23]

In their zeal for championing the virtues of scientific drug development, some cocaine advocates suggested that the therapeutic application of the drug might be guided entirely by laboratory research. In practice, although the new philosophy of drug development certainly supported and encouraged the use of cocaine, many physicians continued to rely on their own clinical experience and personal experimentation. The new research ideology and rhetoric of modernity must, therefore, be joined to an examination of actual medical practice.

Cocaine in Medical Practice

The work of Koller inspired numerous American physicians to experiment with cocaine not only as a surgical anesthetic but also in general medical practice. Subsequent generations remembered Koller less for his pioneering research than as the person who opened Pandora's box by popularizing cocaine. During the decade after Koller's breakthrough, however, cocaine remained confined to medical practice in a variety of therapeutic guises.

Cocaine and Surgery

Before the use of cocaine as a local anesthetic, physicians could choose only from general anesthetics, such as chloroform or ether, or no anesthetic at all. Ether, a relatively new drug, had been introduced in the United States in the 1840s; and although it was certainly appropriate in a variety of operations, it was of little use in others. Cocaine allowed physicians to perform delicate operations that were difficult under general anesthetics, particularly in cases in which reactions such as retching and vomiting would cause uncontrollable movement in the patient. By eliminating these difficulties, the use of cocaine as a topical anesthetic allowed the surgeon greater control.[24]

Cocaine also allowed patients to remain awake and in control. Before the introduction of cocaine, operations in which the patient was required to assist the manipulations of the physician such as in operations on the eye and the throat, were performed with great difficulty, if at all. Before cocaine, such operations, if attempted, were excruciating for the patient and understandably difficult for the surgeon. In October 1884, Le Roy Pope Walker wrote of a young female patient who had unsuccessful surgery performed without ether. According to his account, the pain was so great during this first operation that "a dozen young doctors could scarcely hold her." She came to Walker, "prepared to take ether, even at the risk of her life." Walker performed the operation successfully with cocaine, and the young woman felt no pain. The *Virginia Medical Monthly* reported that "to the specialist, cocaine finds its greatest triumphs in the operation for cataract and irridectomy. It seems almost incredible that a patient can calmly look on and see every motion of the operator on the other." When the patient was required to remain conscious, cocaine provided an anesthetic that would free the patient from pain and suffering and allow the physician to work without resistance.[25]

Cocaine broadened the base of potential candidates for surgery by allowing physicians to operate on previously unacceptable subjects. Although general anesthesia had made certain operations easier, operating under anesthesia still required physicians to make prior judgments about a patient's fitness for surgery. Generally speaking, candidates were required to be of a strong constitution, with no predisposition toward "nervousness."[26] Walker, in a report of fourteen surgical cases, recorded that eight of the fourteen were either "very nervous" or had been resisting medical interference before the use of cocaine. Two others were small children. In each case, the operations were performed without pain or discomfort and with "little resistance." According to Martin Pernick, with the advent of cocaine in 1884 and 1885, "anesthetists began to concentrate more on tailoring the choice of anesthetic to suit the patient, instead of selecting those patients best suited to anesthesia."[27]

The practice of ophthalmologist T. R. Pooley illustrates the changes brought on by the advent of cocaine. Pooley, who practiced in New York, first employed cocaine in a surgical procedure on October 17, 1884, only days after word of Koller's work appeared in the United States. Before cocaine, eye operations were dangerously unpredictable, as in the case of "a very pusillanimous old man" from whom Pooley attempted to remove a cataract. Operating without ether, Pooley claimed that the elderly patient's "bad behavior came near to costing him his eye" as the patient had moved while Pooley's knife was near the eye, causing some secondary damage to the cornea. After Pooley adopted the use of cocaine, one of his first patients was the same elderly gentleman, who although "very apprehensive of pain" felt nothing during a successful operation. Another patient, who had a splinter of wood driven into the eye, had cocaine applied to the eye and the splinter removed. According to Pooley, "With any except the most heroic of subjects such an operation could hardly have been performed without the use of ether." Pooley observed that cocaine could "enable one to make all such operations as these with ease, and only requires the minimum exhibition of courage."[28] Eye operations of these kinds began to be viewed as suitable for all but the weakest of character and constitution.

Cocaine also proved useful in nose and throat surgery, extremely difficult to conduct without anesthetics but nearly impossible *with* general anesthetics. According to William Moore in late 1884, "in the surgery of the pharynx and larynx, above all other parts, it [cocaine] was an agent surpassing any hitherto known, for with general anesthesia the futility of operations on these passages was well known, as the patient's consciousness was needed to aid in the necessary manipulations," yet with cocaine "we could pick out a tumor from the larynx with as much ease as a cork out of a bottle."[29] Laryngologist William Chapman Jarvis reported that a patient who had been suffering from a deviated septum was unable to allow the doctor to touch the area with his instruments. After an application of cocaine solution, the patient not only allowed Jarvis to probe the area but to remove the deviated cartilage as well. According to Jarvis, "the patient could with difficulty find words to express his profound sense of satisfaction." As the ophthalmologists had found, cocaine allowed Jarvis to expand his base of patients for surgery. A young female patient, for example, "did not possess one particle of fortitude, causing a great deal of trouble by her persistent crying, and in spite of every precaution for her comfort she proved herself to be one of the most intractable patients I ever had to contend with." Nevertheless, when he treated her with cocaine, Jarvis was able to operate on her nose without difficulty.[30]

Physicians also employed cocaine in nonsurgical procedures that required assessment of sensitive areas. Physicians were able to examine patients who had painful throat conditions by spraying a cocaine solution into the throat. Both urethral and gynecological exams were also aided by applications of cocaine.

Other American researchers expanded the role of cocaine in surgery beyond its use as a local anesthetic. Experiments conducted by William Halsted (later the first professor of surgery at the Johns Hopkins University School of Medicine) pioneered the use of cocaine as the first nerve block anesthetic. Another American surgeon, J. Leonard Corning, employed cocaine in the first successful attempt at nerve trunk anesthesia, although this procedure was not integrated into regular surgical practice for several years.

Cocaine as Tonic and Stimulant

The uses of cocaine in general medicine reflected the belief that the drug was highly effective against "nervous" disease. Consequently, neurologists conducted much of the important cocaine research. In 1884, neurology was still a relatively small medical specialty in the United States, with the first neurological association organized only nine years earlier. Nevertheless, the leading figures in neurology were highly influential in the profession at large, and their diagnoses and theories helped shape medical practice.

In addition to treating organic diseases of the nervous system, neurologists shared a responsibility for managing "nervous" diseases, many of which would be considered neuroses of some sort today or would have an unrelated physical cause. The nineteenth-century practice of psychiatry, which might have been expected to deal with so-called nervous diseases, was instead confined to the treatment of insanity. So, while the psychiatrist practiced in asylums, the neurologist treated patients with relatively minor complaints, setting the stage for the prominent role of neurologists in the development of psychotherapy.[31]

Before the development of modern psychotherapy, however, the most important neurological concept was neurasthenia. Discovered by American neurologist George Miller Beard, neurasthenia was an important step in the "evolution of nervousness." The concept identified a series of conditions as products of nervousness in progressively more serious forms: nervous dyspepsia, headache, nearsightedness, chorea, sleeplessness, hay fever, hypochondria, hysteria, neurasthenia, inebriety, epilepsy, and insanity. Neurasthenia was both a cause of nervous disease as well as an effect. The conditions linked to nervousness were poorly understood, and "nervousness" offered a satisfying and comprehensive explanation.[32]

What caused nervousness? Most American physicians attributed it to the stresses and strains caused by a rapidly changing and growing industrial society. These were said to be particularly acute among brain workers, whose exhausting work habits "depleted" their nerves. As William Searle (whose advocacy of coca has already been noted) described the problem, it was largely a matter of overstimulation. Searle singled out "our business and professional men" as those for whom the danger was greatest. Although the neurasthenia diagnosis eventually broadened to include working-class patients, throughout the 1880s it remained primarily a disorder afflicting the middle and upper classes, both men and women.[33]

Because nervousness had at least some physical basis, drug therapy came to be part of the treatment. After 1884, neurologists adopted cocaine for nervous patients, the rationale being that if cocaine could act with such powerful effect on the nerves during surgical procedures, it seemed to follow that it might also restore debilitated nerves.

Ironically, the use of cocaine in the treatment of nervous disease borrowed heavily from the once-discredited claims for its tonic and strengthening effects. George Beard, who died in 1883 before the start of widespread cocaine use, noted these claims in his 1880 text, *A Practical Treatise on Nervous Exhaustion*. Although not a champion of coca, the inventor of neurasthenia wrote, "The value of coca . . . is erroneously exaggerated in the stock anecdotes that appear . . . but it has, without doubt, a special and most interesting sustaining and tonic power. It relieves the pain and uneasiness that follow over-exertion, and the peculiar distress that comes from sleepless nights, for which purpose, I may say, caffeine may also be used." In 1886, D. R. Brower of Chicago reported that although he had been using cocaine for only one year, he had employed coca in his practice since 1880 as a brain stimulant and to treat opium addiction, melancholia, and neurasthenia.[34]

Research into the physiological action of cocaine seemed to confirm its utility in the area of nervous disease. In his textbook on materia medica, H. C. Wood claimed that "the most susceptible portion of the body to the action of cocaine is the cerebrum."[35] The work of European physicians supported the work of American researchers. Sigmund Freud, at the time a young neurologist, found inspiration on coca while reading early reports published in the *Therapeutic Gazette*. In his first published study, Freud suggested that the nerve-strengthening properties of cocaine might prove useful in treating nervous disease. Freud began by observing that psychiatrists already had many drugs available which could be used to sedate patients. Such drugs, he felt, reduced the "excitation" of the nerve centers. What psychiatrists lacked, Freud wrote, were drugs that could *increase* the functioning of nerve centers. Freud believed that cocaine was such a drug and urged its adoption in the treatment of hypochondria, hysteria, and melancholy.[36]

Based on this research and their own clinical experience, physicians employed cocaine as a tonic for the nerves. One extension of this was the use of cocaine to support and strengthen patients with serious diseases. Patients with tuberculosis, cholera, syphilis, and yellow fever all received cocaine. The *Philadelphia Medical Times* reported that coca was an effective "stimulant, tonic, and restorative to the system in the treatment of various diseases marked by debility and exhaustion."[37]

Some physicians also suspected that cocaine might enhance mental performance and ability. Medical reports included references to users being able to read for hours at a time or to write at great length. A physician in Portland, Maine, took cocaine for sleeplessness and found that he "felt wide awake in a moment and was able to read understandingly a very abstruse book."[38] Many published reports were, in fact, descriptions of self-experimentation among physicians, most of which concluded that cocaine made "the flow of thought more easy and the reasoning power more vigorous" or fostered "a keenness of perception and a mental vigor greater than normal."[39] Brower aptly summarized medical opinion in 1886, stating that cocaine was "the most certain and agreeable of mental stimulants."[40]

Besides allowing brain work to be performed more readily, cocaine seemed to relieve the stress and mild depression that might lead to more serious nervous disease. A doctor who "had the blues" reported that smoking coca leaf cigars after dinner had the effect of dispelling his depression.[41] A female patient suffering from exhaustion and confined to her bed for a year was given a coca preparation and almost immediately found her spirits restored "and promises to be soon restored to her former condition of health."[42]

In more serious cases such as melancholia, neurologists also looked for possible therapeutic benefit in cocaine. Former surgeon general and leading neurologist William Hammond reported to the New York Neurological Society the successful treatment of three cases of melancholia in "women who refused to speak." According to Hammond, "the injections of cocaine had overcome the prolonged silence." To the American Neurological Society in 1885, Jerome Baudy described how he "frequently witnessed, the morose, silent, taciturn patient, a prey to the most profound grief or sadness, recover his normal self, begin to talk about his case and wonder how he could ever have experienced such gloomy ideas."[43]

Cocaine never wholly replaced preparations of coca as the tonic of choice in medical practice. Not all the coca imported into the United States went into cocaine manufacture; pharmaceutical companies produced many coca preparations, often in combination with traditional "tonic" agents such as alcohol, beef extract, iron, quinine, and tea. Thus, physicians might prescribe coca and beef compounds or coca, beef, and iron. By far the most popular combination was coca and wine, which was both palatable and potent. As Grant suffered through the final stages of his terminal cancer, his weakness and fatigue led Douglas to try to restore some of the general's vitality with a coca wine.[44]

As a tonic and a brain stimulant, coca preparations held the most prominent place. In an 1893 survey of Philadelphia physicians, Lewis Adler found that of ten physicians who had employed cocaine or coca as a tonic or mental stimulant, six used coca exclusively. Those who employed cocaine recommended small doses, ranging from 1 to 2 grains daily. Although noted Philadelphia physician Solomon Solis-Cohen used cocaine as a physical stimulant, and especially as a cardiac stimulant, as a tonic he preferred "the coca-leaf, in the form of a reliable fluid extract, alcoholic or aqueous. It seems to contain other principles and to differ from cocaine in its action, almost as opium differs from morphine, or cinchona from quinine." Of the five others who employed coca, three used no cocaine at all, and two others prescribed cocaine in other conditions.[45]

W. Golden Mortimer surveyed physicians in 1898 and 1899 regarding coca in medical practice, and the results show that coca appeared most often as a tonic and stimulant. Based on responses from 369 physicians nationwide, Mortimer found the most prominent therapeutic uses were in cases of debility (141 responses), exhaustion (133), neurasthenia (124), and overwork (106). Although these results suggest only that those who employed coca sought its tonic and stimulant benefits, the medical literature does offer some compelling evidence that those desiring a tonic and stimulant utilized coca more often than cocaine.

Cocaine in the Treatment of Opiate Addiction

By 1884, physicians had identified the phenomenon of opiate addiction as a substantial national problem. The rate of opiate addiction may well have been at its highest in the late nineteenth century.[46] Changes in the medical use of opiates accounted for much of the increased prevalence of addiction. These changes involved a long-term shift away from milder forms of opiates (such as laudanum or Dover's powder) toward morphine as well as the popularization of the hypodermic syringe in the 1870s. The hypodermic, in particular, gave physicians a potent way to relieve pain with morphine and gave opiate users a powerful drug experience.[47] Most physicians recognized their responsibility for the epidemic and stressed the importance of trying to treat the opiate addict.

Physicians hardly had to seek out opiate addicts for treatment; instead, they were confronted by addicts desperate to stop using opiates or equally desperate for a continued supply. One young addict sought a cure from his doctor by declaring he "would sooner be dead than live the life of slavery much longer." Another doctor offered the typical case of "Mr. X.Y.," who had "begun using morphine in 1877 for lumbago, and had reached a dose of twenty-five grs. as a maximum, three to four times a day." Mr. X.Y.'s "nervous depression became so great that he could not hold his pen, or button his shirt, or handle knife and fork at breakfast, without taking his usual dose directly after rising." With such a large and desperate market, countless private sanitariums, patent medicines, and traveling quacks claimed they could cure addiction.[48]

As the problem of opiate addiction grew, so did the number of cures available to the public. An inebriety movement in medicine emerged and included a national organization and journal. Private institutions appeared in every state, ready to offer addicts a sure cure. Some, like the Keeley Institute of Illinois, grew into national chains of addiction treatment centers. Alongside the institutions, a host of mail order and over-the-counter preparations promised to break the dependence on opiates. Most products and therapies were as useless as they were popular. But professional medical authority was weak, and nowhere was this more obvious than the marketplace for addiction treatment.

Cocaine offered physicians the possibility of retaining addicts as patients and competing with therapeutic alternatives. This approach to treating opiate addiction had first been suggested by the coca enthusiasts, who promoted the administration of a stimulant during the withdrawal of opiates.[49] Indeed, Sigmund Freud's interest in this area reflected his reading of these early articles. Freud came close to calling cocaine a specific cure for morphine addiction, believing its action not only provided stimulation and support during withdrawal but was directly antagonistic to the physiological effects of morphine.[50] More often, physicians saw cocaine as a tool for overcoming the difficulties of opiate withdrawal. Because getting an addict through the withdrawal period represented the most immediate obstacle to treatment, this was a considerable benefit.

The emerging definition of addiction as a manifestation of nervous disease reinforced the view that cocaine was potentially helpful in treating opiate dependence. Neurasthenia and nervousness helped doctors explain why some patients fell victim to addiction while others appeared to avoid serious harm. Beard, for example, located inebriety between neurasthenia and insanity on the scale of nervous disorders[51]; therefore, cocaine might palliate the harsher symptoms of withdrawal while attacking the underlying nervousness that predisposed the patient toward addiction.

The initial response of addicts to cocaine treatment seemed encouraging. A detailed account by physician J. T. Whittaker highlighted the potential of cocaine for reducing treatment frustrations. In 1885, a young patient of Whittaker's checked into the Good Samaritan Hospital in Cincinnati after several failed attempts at home to stop her use of morphine. The discomfort of withdrawal was enough to send her climbing out through the hospital window on sheets tied together. She was found across the street pounding on the door of a neighboring drugstore to awaken the clerk. After a short period of sobriety, the young woman returned to morphine. In desperation, she went back to Dr. Whittaker and reentered the hospital. In return, Dr. Whittaker had to promise that he "would prevent any undue suffering — anything that approached her previous experience — by the use of a sufficient quantity of morphia." In hopes of keeping his promise, Whittaker gave her repeated injections of cocaine during her first two days in the hospital. After this, by some continued use of cocaine, the patient no longer used morphine and, according to Whittaker "was herself persuaded . . . that she had won such an easy victory by the use of the injections of cocaine."[52]

Almost from the start, however, the medical profession was divided on the benefits of coca or cocaine in the treatment of addiction. Freud is the best known advocate of this form of treatment, but similar recommendations were surprisingly scarce in the American medical literature. Where physicians did employ cocaine, recommended doses were slightly higher than in typical cocaine treatments of nervous disease, 0.5 to 2 grains, taken three to four times daily. The most common treatment plan involved gradually reducing an addict's dose of opium or morphine and substituting frequent (and sometimes increasing) doses of cocaine. The gradual reduction treatment was spread out over varying lengths of time, usually about a week. At this point, most physicians urged their patients to discontinue cocaine. A smaller number encouraged continued use whenever a patient felt the desire for opiates.

The physicians who could successfully "cure" patients of their addiction found real professional rewards. Patients showed remarkably positive physical changes, reinforcing the notion of the reinvigorating properties of cocaine. Physicians appreciated the gratitude of patients who had won their "easy victories" over opiates. Of course, some patients continued to employ cocaine on their own, but few contemplated the possibility of cocaine addiction disrupting their lives even more surely than opiate addiction.

Cocaine and Hay Fever

Among the most common medical applications of cocaine were those that dealt with irritation of the sinuses. The extensive use of cocaine in surgical procedures in the nasal passages created an awareness of its vasoconstrictive properties, which could open swollen sinus passages and relieve the suffering of sinus irritation caused by colds and hay fever. In an article published in the *Medical Record* of November 15, 1884, Francke Bosworth described the contraction in the mucous membrane which followed an application of cocaine in solution. Bosworth reported the results of forty cases he had already treated, including twenty-seven cases of swollen sinuses, seven cases of ordinary head colds, four cases of swollen nasal polyps, and two cases of hay fever. Bosworth proclaimed that "there is no longer any excuse for anyone suffering from a cold in the head." This early work was cited extensively in the seventh edition (1889) of H. C. Wood's standard medical reference text, *Therapeutics: Its Principles and Practice.*[53]

As they had with neurasthenia and opiate addiction, late-nineteenth-century physicians often linked diseases such as hay fever, asthma, catarrh, rose colds, and coryza in some way to diseases of the nervous system or "neuroses of the respiratory system." This explained why, according to Seth Bishop, "the class of people who suffer from this affection are the nervous, brain-working type, instead of the phlegmatic, slow-going kind, who may be more exposed to the pollen of the field or the dust of the work-shop and street, but whose minds are strangers to the nervous stimulation and mental tension of the professional man."[54]

Not everyone agreed with the idea that hay fever was of nervous origin, of course, but Roberts Bartholow summarized the logic of those who did. Bartholow observed that every person in a given community was exposed to the same "foreign bodies" in the air. Thus, he reasoned, those who suffered from hay fever must be uniquely susceptible to these irritants. Further, what was unique to hay fever sufferers was a "peculiar type of nervous system." By acting upon the nerves, cocaine could actually cure this common condition. Bartholow praised cocaine, concluding that "in various neuroses of the respiratory organs, asthma, whooping-cough, singultus, etc. there can be no doubt respecting its curative power."[55]

Doctors were again divided over the question of whether cocaine was a cure or a palliative. Some, such as Bartholow, had "no doubt" that cocaine could cure. Most disagreed, observing the effects of cocaine to be temporary and concluding that cocaine promised only short-term relief of symptoms. Even physicians who found cocaine to be "merely" a palliative, however, recommended its use, noting that it "gave great comfort" to those who would otherwise be "obliged to flee to hay fever resorts." In *Cocaine in Hay Fever*, Seth Bishop concluded that it was "highly improbable that cocaine will ever prove to be a cure for hay fever," yet "as a palliative it acts like magic in some cases."[56]

The treatment of respiratory complaints involved cocaine almost to the exclusion of coca because of the vasoconstricting effects of cocaine, which oral-dosage coca preparations could not provide. Mortimer's survey of coca use revealed that only 30 of the 369 physicians employed coca in asthma whereas 32 used it for the lungs. None of Mortimer's respondents employed coca for colds, hay fever, or sinus ailments.[57] Cocaine, on the other hand, had a consistent effect on the nasal passages. The physician merely had to instruct patients to self-administer a nasal spray or snuff whenever they desired relief.[58] There was less resistance to prescribing higher doses because many regarded sprays and snuffs as topical applications rather than internal medicine. As the price of cocaine fell, doctors found sniffing cocaine in its powdered form affordable and effective.[59]

While the medical community debated whether to classify cocaine as a cure or a palliative, many practitioners appeared willing to endorse its use in either case. Cocaine worked and could be self-administered easily. Because this usage required cocaine rather than coca, patients were not given the relatively low dosage obtained through coca or coca products; and because the action of cocaine was only temporary, patients were encouraged to make frequent use of it as the symptoms of a cold or hay fever returned.

The medical use of cocaine has often been described as "faddish," which conveys a sense of medical ignorance and implies a failure to evaluate the new drug critically and objectively.[60] Still other accounts suggest that the therapeutic applications of cocaine were merely a convenient cover for those who wished to enjoy its pleasurable effects surreptitiously. These charges, which almost certainly would have surprised the physicians of the late nineteenth century, are not well supported by the historical evidence.

To be sure, many of the earliest reports in medical journals tended to overpraise the new drug, especially those reports that sought to use cocaine to illustrate the promise of modern laboratory research and physiological therapeutics. But too close a focus on these reports alone almost surely results in an exaggerated picture of the medical response. In practice, physicians limited coca or cocaine to several common applications: as an anesthetic, a tonic, and a sinus remedy. The amounts administered or prescribed in its use as a tonic, far from appearing indiscriminate, appear to have been fairly conservative. The Philadelphia physicians surveyed by Adler reported the use of ⅛ to 1 grain (8–65 milligrams) of cocaine, several times daily, for short terms.[61]

In only two specific instances does the contention that cocaine prescription was indiscriminate seem even partly accurate. First, in the treatment of opiate addiction, cocaine sometimes served as a substitute for morphine or opium with little thought to the effects of its long-term use, particularly when physicians supplied addicts with cocaine and told them to employ it whenever the craving for opiates returned. Yet even in the treatment of addiction, the tremendous diversity of medical practice makes easy generalizations difficult. The second, and more egregious, area of indiscriminate cocaine prescription was in the treatment of asthma and hay fever. Here, physicians adopted cocaine to the exclusion of coca preparations and recommended much higher doses over longer periods of time while frankly acknowledging that its effect was only temporary and palliative.

The adoption of cocaine in medical practice set the stage for its subsequent popularization; indeed, there is little reason to believe that widespread cocaine consumption would have occurred otherwise. Yet the role of medical professionals was hardly that of zealous missionaries. Taken together, the accounts of therapeutic practice suggest instead the need to take seriously the context of nineteenth-century medicine and the role of physicians in defining the earliest boundaries of acceptable cocaine consumption.

TWO

Debating the Dangers of Cocaine

The Medical Era, 1885–1895

The "medical era" of cocaine use began with Koller's landmark research in 1884 and lasted for about a decade. During that time, physicians controlled much of the cocaine supply. Little explicitly nonmedical consumption existed; even purchases for personal, nonmedical use most often had their origins in medical practice. As the medical profession elevated cocaine from obscurity to a drug of first choice, its members were also engaged in the first serious discussions of the safety and overuse of the drug.

The evidence of early medical praise for the benefits of cocaine and the subsequent concerns over its dangers can be misread as a simple progression from the former to the latter.[1] Historical evidence suggests that even as medical opinion came to identify some potential dangers, many physicians continued to endorse the therapeutic advantages of cocaine in their practices. Firmly believing that any danger associated with cocaine could be minimized by limiting its use to skilled professionals, most physicians neither wholly rejected nor wholly embraced cocaine. They did, however, raise serious concerns about two important dangers: "cocaine poisoning" and the creation of the "cocaine habit."[2] Rather than calling for the elimination of cocaine, most physicians advocated strict medical control and conservative use to avoid an expansion of either problem.

The fear of cocaine poisoning, which was as great as the fear of the cocaine habit, figured prominently in the self-regulation of medical practice. The concept of poisoning incorporated a broad range of reactions, including purely toxic ones such as cardiac arrhythmia or convulsions as well as strange behavioral effects caused by the euphoriant or stimulant actions of the drug and even a patient's fearful response to unfamiliar or unpleasant effects.

The concept of a cocaine habit also appeared in the months after the initial burst of medical enthusiasm. Although a minority of physicians took the position that the cocaine habit did not exist, a consensus quickly emerged that the drug could create uncontrollable cravings that led to self-destructive patterns of use. This medical consensus distinguished the cocaine habit from opiate addiction, concluding that the overuse of cocaine originated from different impulses (a "habit of the mind") and produced starkly different physical and behavioral symptoms. Indeed, the seductiveness of cocaine encouraged the view that it was the worst drug to place in the hands of the general public.

In the absence of legal regulation of the drug supply or formal professional controls over therapeutic practice, the task of defining "safe" and "legitimate" use fell to individual physicians. Most determined that controlling their own application of the drug would mitigate the serious problems associated with either cocaine poisoning or the cocaine habit. Two aspects of this problem definition led physicians to conclude that such control was possible. First, the cocaine habit was thought to be largely a result of overprescription. What doctors had caused, they reasoned, they might also control merely by strengthening their role as gatekeepers to the nation's drug supply. Second, poisoning and habitual use were thought to depend upon individual patient idiosyncrasy. Identifying potential victims would allow physicians to prescribe cocaine freely to everyone else. The concept that some patients might be more vulnerable to the dangers of cocaine also prompted generalizations based on the race, class, and ethnicity of the user. The middle-class demographic profile of the typical cocaine habitué in this era of medical use did not promote panicked or punitive responses from physicians. The medical-era belief that therapeutic use could continue without presenting a social problem is significant; not until the social profile of the cocaine user changed would physicians lead the fight for legal control.

Cocaine Poisoning

Given the extent of medical and social concerns over cocaine abuse today, it may seem surprising that concerns over poisoning dominated the medical era. Reports of cocaine poisoning appeared in the medical literature almost immediately. Reactions included a variety of unpleasant and frightening symptoms. Some reports even suggested that in large doses, death could result.

The response of the medical profession to cocaine poisoning can best be described as uncertain. Some physicians abandoned cocaine because of its potential toxicity; others discounted the danger entirely. Most physicians, however, found cause for concern in reports of adverse reactions to cocaine and chose to employ it conservatively to avoid problems.

The majority of reported cases of cocaine poisoning involved its use as a local anesthetic. Illustrative of this pattern is the work of J. B. Mattison. In 1887, Mattison presented sixty-eight cases in which patients suffered negative reactions to cocaine. Of the sixty-eight reports, fifty involved the use of cocaine as a local anesthetic.[3] The reasons for the large numbers of surgical cases are not entirely clear, but there are several likely explanations. One is the high dosage involved in producing anesthesia compared with lower dosages in other common therapeutic applications.[4] Another reason is the use of cocaine by hypodermic injection in many surgical cases, which may have increased the rapidity with which cocaine was absorbed, thus causing more severe reactions. Because of the higher risk involved in the surgical uses of cocaine, the few reported deaths from cocaine poisoning involved surgical cases.[5]

Deaths from cocaine were exceedingly rare, but other symptoms of cocaine poisoning were far more common. An early report in the *Therapeutic Gazette* listed the following symptoms: "general intoxication, nausea, and vomiting, lasting an entire day, stumbling gait, syncope (cerebral anemia?), pallor and sweating, loss of consciousness, and convulsions."[6] One physician described the serious symptoms of cocaine poisoning, including what appeared to be temporary paralysis and wryly noted that ever since, when employing cocaine "a vision arises before me of this patient as she appeared with the whole body apparently paralyzed, except her tongue . . . this unruly member continually uttering words of reproach to me for the helpless and hopeless condition in which I had placed all the other members, gave me a sensation that I have no desire to experience again."[7]

Other reactions, although considerably less serious, concerned both doctor and patient. A New Jersey physician, J. W. Stickler, described three experiences with cocaine poisoning. In one instance, an injection of cocaine caused a patient's face to "swell up like a balloon." A similar application to a second patient's finger likewise caused it to swell. In the third case, a patient who took 9 grains of cocaine for a toothache could not sleep even after Stickler administered 20 grains of chloral hydrate and a teaspoonful of laudanum.[8] Another physician concluded that "these are the things which tend to frighten us in the use of cocaine."[9]

Along with the physical reactions to cocaine came other reports of strange mental reactions. An early experiment by M. D. Hoge on a colleague suggested the potential for cocaine to evoke strange or inappropriate behavior. After taking 3 grains (194 milligrams) internally, Hoge's colleague described his feeling as "glorious all over the body, with stimulating waves rushing through his limbs." After the administration of another 4 grains (295 milligrams) of cocaine over the next hour, Hoge reported that his colleague was "very talkative; the talk is not connected, but a repetition of the same idea over and over because words fail to express the delightful sensations." After a third hour, with no more cocaine, his colleague was "sober, but feels foolish."[10]

D. S. Booth, surgeon in charge at the Great Northern Railroad Hospital in Texas, reported an unusual experience after the injection of cocaine in the urethra. Booth gave his patient a cocaine solution, with instructions to inject half. The patient, "led by the general belief that if a 'little does good more will do better'," injected the whole amount. The patient's own account of the experience suggests its unusual character:

> Having injected the cocaine solution, I at once lay down on the bed, retaining the solution in the urethra for about fifteen minutes. In about ten minutes I experienced a soothing sensation which soon permeated my whole frame, making me feel as though I had neither trouble nor care. This lasted about ten minutes, when an extraordinary sense of abundant vitality and pent-up energy seized me, causing me to get up from bed with a strong desire for violent exercise. Three quarters of an hour must have elapsed, of which I have hardly any recollection. I have a dim remembrance of standing out in the yard, trying to pass water, a remembrance which must be materially assisted by the fact that excruciating pain accompanied the effort. I do not recollect whether I succeeded in making water or not, though I am told I did. The next thing I distinctly remember is sitting on the front steps, though even then I was not able to fix my mind on any one thing, my ideas seeming to get all mixed up. After a short while my brain seemed to clear up, leaving me with a severe headache. On getting up the next morning I felt as well as if nothing had occurred.[11]

Other physicians experienced the same or similar difficulties with cocaine. Mattison reported a case in which a patient "became maniacal, and under the delusion that he had been attacked by a robber, sprang from his seat, seized the doctor by the throat and began to beat him."[12] A dentist wrote to the *Medical Brief* reporting the case of a "well-developed young girl" sixteen years old brought to his office for a tooth extraction. To lessen the pain of the operation, the doctor injected cocaine into her gums. As he was about to remove the tooth, the patient "gently closed her eyes and seemed to undergo a paroxysm of the most intense pleasurable excitement, accompanying her actions by words uttered in a half delirious manner, that fairly astounded me." The dentist was "very much puzzled" by the patient's reaction, concluding that it was most likely an aphrodisiac quality of cocaine which caused the behavior.[13]

Although physicians understood that cocaine sometimes produced these responses, they could not predict when they would occur or in whom. Moreover, these reactions seemed to occur at different dosages, frustrating physicians who sought to determine an assuredly "safe" level. Because the timing of these reactions was unpredictable, some of the more unusual responses were enough to merit serious concern.

In an 1899 presentation to the Philadelphia Neurological Society, J. Chalmers DaCosta related two cases of his own which were unusual and unexpected. The first patient was given 1.25 grains of cocaine to inject into the urethra. Not long after doing so, the patient experienced marked physical responses to the cocaine, including temporary unconsciousness. What followed were "hallucinations of sight and hearing of an agreeable nature," as DaCosta described them,

> he would answer when spoken to, but could not maintain a thread of conversation, and when left to himself was concentrated on his own ideas, which flowed in a torrent, now grave, now gay, now majestic, now amusing. This condition was one of intellectual brilliancy. He quoted poetry, oratory, and philosophy (being a particularly well educated man, and a writer himself of some attainments). He gave portions of "Locksley Hall," with excellent effect, and wept as he recited Keats' "Ode to A Nightingale." When told that he had fainted while grabbing his penis, and asked what would have been said by his friends had he died in that attitude, he responded, "The ruling passion is strong in death."

In an unsurprising turn of events, that patient repeated the experiment again at his home "with the result of alarming his family to a terrible extent." As unsettling as this experience may have been for DaCosta, the second reported case was surely more so. After administering an injection of cocaine in the urethra of the first patient's twenty-year-old brother, DaCosta reported that the patient "staggered about the office, upset chairs, aimed blows at me, and, with indistinct articulation, declared that I wanted to kill him." The patient awoke the next morning "very penitent" but with little memory of what had occurred.[14]

The discussion among the members of the Philadelphia Neurological Society which followed DaCosta's presentation revealed uncertainty about the reported cases. Dr. Francis X. Dercum suggested that perhaps the urethra was especially sensitive to cocaine because he had never observed similar symptoms in his administration of it in other areas. Two other physicians seconded this view, although E. N. Brush noted that cocaine administered to melancholic patients produced "laughter in some, and a talkative state." DaCosta concluded by noting the confused state of the subject: "The dangerous dose therefore seems to be some-where between the wide extremes of 0.10 grain (6 milligrams) and 32 grains (2,074 milligrams), but exactly where is hard to tell."[15]

Amid the confusion, some concluded that cocaine had no toxic effect at all. Although these physicians were never in the majority, they do highlight the ab-sence of general consensus. When D. R. Brower reported some "alarming" cases of collapse from cocaine poisoning to the Chicago Medical Society in 1886, col-leagues voiced skepticism that such results could be attributed to the drug. One noted the inclusion of a case in Brower's report in which a patient had lost con-sciousness after the injection of 0.8 gram of cocaine and said he "doubted very much whether the bad effects were due to cocaine," noting that "we get the same effect in many patients by injecting water, or by showing them the hypodermic syringe." He concluded that it "was simply a fainting fit."[16]

The enduring skepticism showed up in a 1903 presentation to the San Fran-cisco Society of Eye, Ear, Nose, and Throat Surgeons in which Dr. Robert Cohn presented the details of a cocaine-poisoning case. In this instance, Cohn applied cocaine to a surgical patient's nose. As Cohn completed the operation to remove a bone spur from the septum, the patient turned pale and complained of dizzi-ness. The patient collapsed, experienced rapid breathing, and his pulse rate ran as high as 160. For three hours the patient "hovered between life and death," and, according to Cohn, "we thought every minute we would lose him." The patient recovered, and Cohn presented his experience to the surgical society. Louis Deane responded by suggesting that "there are few of us who can not state sim-ilar cases of a much milder character, the result of mere aural or nasal application where no anesthetic was used." Another agreed with Deane, suggesting that "as a rule, I think the collapse is more from the idea of an operation than from the co-cain[e]." Still another thought the collapse was related "to a psychical condition." Although some individuals might be peculiarly susceptible to cocaine, the doc-tors argued, its moderate use was not injurious.[17]

The individual-idiosyncrasy theory compelled even those physicians with no clinical experience with poisoning to be cautious because any patient might sud-denly succumb.[18] By employing cocaine conservatively, the profession hoped to avoid an increase in negative reactions and retain a valuable remedy. Physician self-reports revealed a pattern of small dosages, so reports of cocaine poisoning reinforced already conservative tendencies. W. Sheppegrell urged the Orleans Parish Medical Society, for example, not to consider cocaine "an unalloyed bless-ing" and advocated greater attention to the quantity of cocaine administered be-cause lower amounts "would be less likely to develop toxic symptoms" than higher doses.[19]

Lewis Adler's survey of Philadelphia physicians found many keeping dosages low to avoid cocaine poisoning even though fewer than one in five reported previous experience with toxic reactions. Frederick P. Henry employed cocaine frequently in cases of "nervous dyspepsia" but reported that "the doses in which I use it are small, rarely exceeding one-fourth of a grain, and it is probably for this reason that I have not seen in my own practice any toxic effects from the internal administration of the drug." Charles Hay also reported freedom from toxic effects in the treatment of melancholia by limiting doses to 0.24 grain (16 milligrams).[20]

An earlier survey by Adler of Philadelphia physicians who employed cocaine in minor surgery revealed the same concerns over modifying cocaine use to avoid toxic reactions. Reflecting the prevalence of poisoning cases in surgery, slightly more than one in four reported actual experience with poisoning. Thomas Morton described the utility of cocaine in operations on the eye, examinations of the larynx, and in treatment of painful skin conditions. Morton reported that he would no longer apply cocaine in the urethra, however, citing the "great danger" that he perceived in this application. Carl Seiler's reply to Adler indicated his belief that by using cotton soaked with cocaine to anesthetize the nose rather than a cocaine spray, he would avoid the "systemic effect of cocaine-poisoning . . . frequently spoken of in the medical journals." Dr. J. Henry C. Simes had the unfortunate experience of a fatal case of cocaine poisoning after a urethral operation, yet he continued to employ the drug. To assure himself of its safety, Simes restricted himself to several "rules" for the administration of cocaine: "Never to use a solution stronger than five per cent. Never to apply it to a mucous membrane when it is abraded, lacerated, or cut. Never to use it hypodermically, if the region cannot be cut off from the general circulation by means of an elastic ligature."[21]

That a drug could be both frightening and valuable was nothing new to nineteenth-century practitioners. Charles Chetwood, a New York physician, acknowledged that physicians who experienced cases of cocaine poisoning felt "something of the same kind of fear of this drug that a person is apt to feel toward a dog by whom they have once been bitten." Chetwood reminded his readers, however, that the use of general anesthetics also resulted in similar numbers of toxic and even fatal reactions. Moreover, Chetwood speculated that "they too, undoubtedly, in their early career, had their 'chapter of accidents.'"[22] Even J. B. Mattison, whose efforts to raise awareness of the potential dangers of cocaine were second to none, placed his concerns in the context of allowing continued use of the drug. To the Kings County Medical Society in 1887, Mattison asserted that his intention was merely to ensure the safe use of a valuable remedy, to "draw the line" so that the toll exacted by "ignorant or incautious using" would not damage the "good repute" of the drug in cases where it would serve physicians well.[23]

In short, fears of cocaine toxicity dampened the enthusiasm of surgeons and general practitioners for its therapeutic application but most certainly did not lead to outright rejection of it. Through careful application of cocaine and low dosages, most physicians in the late nineteenth century hoped to reduce toxic reactions and to continue to use the drug in their practice. This perspective extended to another troubling product of the therapeutic application of cocaine: the cocaine habit.

The Cocaine Habit

By the first months of 1885, medical discussions of the potential dangers of cocaine began to include the possibility of some patients compulsively taking it for its pleasurable effects. Levels of consumption in such instances were often well beyond recommended dosages and were thought to produce a kind of physical and mental deterioration eventually. These individuals were often unwilling or unable to quit using cocaine, even with determined outside intervention. Reflecting the alarm over these early cases, published reports in the medical literature soon began to refer to a "cocaine habit," one not unlike the morphine habit but producing some novel and disturbing effects.

Not every physician agreed that the cocaine habit was real; a few insisted that there was no danger from the use of cocaine, maintaining their opinions in the face of contrary viewpoints and a growing body of case studies. Physicians such as J. T. Whittaker, who treated opiate addicts with doses of cocaine, concluded that "the fear of a cocaine habit is quite ungrounded."[24] The best known of these figures was former surgeon general William Hammond. The *New York Medical Journal* summarized Hammond's comments regarding cocaine and the "so-called cocaine habit," which he "regarded . . . as similar to the tea or coffee habit and unlike the opium habit." Hammond, a frequent consumer of cocaine himself, did not believe that a genuine cocaine habit had ever been demonstrated. Hammond's theory relied in no small part on the absence of an obvious physical dependence on cocaine. Users of cocaine, he argued to his colleagues, could stop at any time if they chose to do so. Hammond's remarks drew praise from J. Leonard Corning, who hoped such comments would put an end to the "morbid fear of cocaine spreading throughout the community."[25]

Hammond's comments have been quoted widely by subsequent generations; indeed, Hammond appears with some prominence in nearly every investigation of the medical era. His denials of the addictive potential of cocaine have been employed as evidence of the ignorance and irresponsibility of the medical profession more generally.[26] The problem with this interpretation is an overreliance on the opinions of a noted physician with very unrepresentative views. A blanket denial of the cocaine habit was never characteristic of medical opinion, at least not after the first several months following Koller's discovery.

Adler's survey showed that only two of twenty responding physicians discounted the possibility of a cocaine habit, and five thought that it occurred only in those already addicted to opiates or alcohol. Most accepted the existence of a cocaine habit without firsthand experience, as with cocaine poisoning. Of the forty-two physicians in Adler's Philadelphia survey, only eleven had treated or even knew of cocaine addicts.[27]

The typical medical-era habitué did not sniff cocaine powder but injected cocaine in solution. Of twenty-eight case studies of cocaine addicts identified in the medical literature, eighteen injected cocaine. Six others sprayed cocaine solution into the nose, and one took cocaine in solution orally. In only two cases did the users sniff cocaine powder. The origins of use were decidedly medical:

Origin of Use	No.
Use in nose (hay fever, etc.)	8
Treatment of addiction	6
Depression/exhaustion	4
Rectal disease	2
Experimental use w/morphine	2
Experimental use	1
Unknown	5

No cases of the cocaine habit resulting from surgery appeared in the medical literature; instead, most cases derived from the application of cocaine in some sort of chronic or recurring condition.[28]

The medical explanation for the cocaine habit emphasized the drug's euphoriant and stimulant effects. One Philadelphia physician who used cocaine as a diuretic suggested to Adler that some applications were simply too enjoyable for patients and that "the patient is apt to want it constantly," concluding with a prediction that, although he had not "as yet seen many cocaine-habitués . . . they are developing, and that we shall have more of them to treat in the future."[29] Another agreed, noting that although he also lacked direct experience with cases of the cocaine habit, "the prolonged use of cocaine has never seemed to me to be justifiable, because in such cases it has always been necessary to increase the dose, and such increase has caused stimulation, which it has seemed to me it was unwise to produce . . . I should certainly fear that its prolonged internal use would lead to the formation of the cocaine-habit."[30]

Physicians knew that the treatment of hay fever and related problems involved a dangerous cycle of short-term relief followed by an inevitable recurrence of symptoms. Some early cases of long-term use produced physical and mental effects that went unexplained initially. James C. Wilson gained some experience with "unsuspected" symptoms such as "restlessness, insomnia, loss of appetite, gastric and intestinal indigestion, and constipation alternating with diarrhea." According to Wilson, these problems "were evidently due to the excessive use of nasal sprays of rather strong solutions of cocaine." In every instance, the discontinuance of the cocaine spray was followed very rapidly by recovery.[31]

The treatment of morphine addiction with cocaine (as well as experimental cocaine use by morphine addicts) led some addicts to conclude that the stimulant effects of cocaine balanced the effects of morphine.[32] These addicts alternated doses of cocaine and morphine or took the first speedballs — cocaine and morphine together. Heine Marks of the St. Louis City Hospital observed that "it was not unusual to find hypodermic morphine users combining cocaine with their preparations, sometimes to the extent of from 12 to 15 grains per day [0.75–1 gram]. The soothing qualities of cocaine are well known to the profession. In most cases the cocaine is added to deaden the pain caused by the frequent use of the hypodermic needle."[33] Such doses seemed extraordinary to the physicians who first described these patterns of use, yet they were common among early cocaine habitués whose daily consumption of cocaine averaged at least a gram per day. One morphine/cocaine user reported in the *Quarterly Journal of Inebriety* employed 20-grain doses, with a daily consumption of 80–120 grains (5.3–7.5 grams).[34]

One addict described his first experience with the combination of cocaine and morphine as the "most exhilarating sensations I have ever known, before or since." He quickly discovered the depression that followed: "at the end of this brief period of ecstasy I fell almost instantly into the depth of a despondency as disheartening as the former had been ravishing. From this horrible gloom I could only be roused by another dose of morphia." He resumed cocaine use about a week later to see how well the drugs would aid him in his writing. His experiment was apparently successful, for his use of each drug continued in increasing doses, an average of about 1 gram of each drug hypodermically per day. Although his use caused little physical discomfort, he found that he "suffered almost constantly from depression, which nothing could remove." After about four months of morphine/cocaine use, he entered a hospital. Looking back on his drug-using career, he recalled that he had "been on the verge of suicide, but never really advanced far enough in that direction to actually begin preparations for self-destruction, though I oftentimes would gladly have welcomed death in any other form."[35]

The readiness with which morphine addicts took up cocaine led the profession to retreat from this therapeutic use of cocaine. Cases of combined use were augmented by many instances in which an opiate addict did in fact reduce or eliminate use of morphine but became dependent on cocaine. Perhaps the most famous case is that of Sigmund Freud's friend and colleague Ernst von Fleischl, whom Freud used as a test case of the ability of cocaine to cure morphine addiction. As scholars have noted, the experiment went awry when Fleischl developed classic symptoms of cocaine abuse, including physical deterioration and psychoses.

Several factors persuaded physicians that the danger of the cocaine habit might potentially be more serious than the habits associated with alcohol or opiates. One factor was the apparent seductiveness of cocaine and the rapidity with which the cocaine habit sometimes appeared. Physicians noted that although the onset of opiate addiction seemed to require use of the drug for an extended period of time, usually in the treatment of some chronic complaint, signs of the cocaine habit could appear soon after the initiation of use. Moreover, cocaine addicts seemed to increase their dosages more rapidly than other drug users. H. G. Brainerd of Los Angeles commented that "once the demand for cocaine is created, the amount required to satisfy that demand must be rapidly increased, — much more rapidly than in the case of any other narcotic with which I am acquainted."[36] Another Los Angeles physician, Robert W. Haynes, wrote that "the cocain[e]-habit, though abandoned much more readily than the morphin[e]-habit, is acquired with much greater facility and insidiousness."[37]

Most disturbing to physicians were the extraordinary euphoric properties of cocaine. Although these properties proved useful in several therapeutic settings, they also suggested to physicians that cocaine was dangerously attractive. In 1896, T. D. Crothers wrote that "cocaine is probably the most agreeable of all narcotics, therefore the most dangerous and alluring."[38] A doctor with the cocaine habit echoed this view, describing his feeling that "every part of the body seems to cry out for a new syringe . . . one syringe self-injected is absolutely sure to produce the fascinating desire for a second."[39]

A second factor in establishing the cocaine habit to be more serious than opiate addiction involved the physical and mental breakdown suffered by heavy users. Nineteenth-century opiate addicts often lived with their addictions for years without seriously impairing their family relations or their ability to work.[40] Because of this, the behavior of those therapeutically addicted to opiates was seldom a cause for concern in the late nineteenth century.[41] Nearly every published case of cocaine addiction, however, mentioned startling physical deterioration and associated behavioral changes. Such changes were made all the more startling by their novelty and the growing recognition that the effects of long-term cocaine use did not seem to match any previously experienced symptoms of opiate addiction.

H. G. Brainerd concluded an 1891 review of the cocaine habit by noting "the rapidity of the mental deterioration . . . Within a few months . . . the character of the cocaine habitué is changed, and he becomes unfitted for business."[42] C. C. Stockard described such changes in a patient he had been treating for opiate addiction but who (unknown to Stockard) had also been using cocaine. As Stockard reduced the doses of morphine, the patient went out and secured a large quantity of cocaine. After several days of use, the patient manifested unmistakable signs of paranoia and was convinced that "the people in the house were watching his actions and were talking about and planning against him . . . the sparrows singing in the street were talking about him, the ticking clock was a telegraph machine of some sort, through which people were communicating about and plotting against him."[43] Stockard ultimately committed the patient to an asylum, where he successfully discontinued use of the drug.

The physical deterioration of users could often be as dramatic as the behavioral changes. Nearly every account of long-term cocaine overuse emphasized moderate to severe weight loss — the appearance of one cocaine-using doctor convinced his friends that he was suffering from tuberculosis. To Charles Bunting, observing the residents of his Home for Intemperate Men, cocaine abuse seemed to transform habitués "into an emaciated, hollow-eyed, bilious-faced, flat-chested, helpless limp of humanity — a very caricature of manhood, with a look like a hunted beast, the shrunken frame trembling."[44]

The third cause for concern over the cocaine habit was the difficulty of producing a "cure." That so many cocaine addicts could not be separated from their drug was hard for physicians to explain. Despite the apparent ease with which cocaine was withdrawn initially, published reports cited the difficulty in achieving permanent cures and noted the frequency of relapse.[45] Among twenty-four early case studies, ten patients reported relapses or failures in treatment, and several others were released as "cured" with no follow-up evaluation. One self-described "cocainist" outlined the problem of breaking away from the drug, using language such as "manic desire," which emphasized psychological rather than physical issues.[46] This powerful attraction, with its attendant perils, convinced many physicians that the cocaine habit was the most dangerous of all.

Defining the Boundaries of "Legitimate" Use

Controlling the troubling problems of the cocaine habit and cocaine poisoning, many physicians argued, meant more careful attention to medical usage. The too-ready distribution of cocaine to the public by overenthusiastic members of the profession created a situation in which patients could easily misuse the drug. Judson Andrews of Erie County, New York, was one of many physicians to conclude that "it is largely to the action of the profession and to the writings in the medical journals that we must attribute the responsibility for the formation of this unfortunate habit."[47] The initial solution to the problem was to encourage the gatekeeping function of the individual practitioner in the hopes that stricter scrutiny might result in fewer negative cases and less "illegitimate" consumption.

Cocaine appeared to be precisely the kind of drug which might prove dangerous in the hands of the general public. Particularly suspect were those instances in which the physician prescribed cocaine to be used as necessary, such as the treatment of hay fever. J. B. Mattison, in his various critical commentaries on the medical use of cocaine, reported numerous cases similar to that of a young Detroit man who consulted his doctor in the summer of 1885 for a "severe and persistent case of hay-fever." Three or four days after having been given a prescription for 8 grains of cocaine, the patient returned to the doctor's office, "his face radiant with the hope that he had at last found a specific [for hay fever] and remarked that "he had felt better the last few days than for a year." After one refilled prescription, the doctor heard no more until November, when a druggist informed him that the young man was using eight dollars of cocaine a week. According to Clark, "the habit had gone too far to be easily eradicated, as the young man went on until he became temporarily insane, had to retire from his business, and be under strict supervision until the craving disappeared, a space of about three months."[48]

The cocaine habit must have been encouraged by the freedom with which physicians directed at least some patients to employ the drug. After an initial application by the physician, patients were directed to provide themselves with a spray atomizer, which they would fill with cocaine solution and use whenever symptoms recurred.[49] Seth Bishop, who recognized the cocaine habit and worried about those times when cocaine use "is not directed and limited by skill," nevertheless developed his own inhaler. He endorsed the inhaler as "simple, effective, and easily practiced even in public assemblages, without making one feel offensively conspicuous."[50]

The treatment of opiate addiction also came under fire for allowing self-administration. Indeed, this method of treating opiate addiction was in rapid decline by 1890. Brower told the Chicago Medical Society that although cocaine surely made withdrawal easier, it should be avoided because it provided the addict "an agent much more rapidly disastrous and destructive to the nutrition of the cerebral convolutions; An agent that will soon sink him to a degradation much lower than is possible with either of the others."[51] In a similar vein, Mattison wrote "to the man who has gone down under opium and who thinks of taking to cocaine in hope of being lifted out of the mire, I would say 'don't,' lest he sink deeper."[52] Even the syringe was criticized as too tempting to be left in the hands of the patient. In an 1898 address to the Atlanta Society of Medicine, C. C. Stockard described the "fascination about the syringe which causes the patient to more rapidly increase the doses taken than when used by the stomach." In such cases, he observed, "the evil consequences are proportionally greater . . . it is only a matter of wonder that this sort of drugging does not kill more rapidly than it does." Stockard concluded his remarks with the suggestion that "the time is not far off" when the government would regulate the sale of drugs likely to be abused.[53]

Self-regulation by physicians often meant keeping dosages small and carefully controlled. In other cases, it meant keeping patients altogether ignorant of the drug being administered. This effort to keep the genie in the bottle was well under way when Adler surveyed physicians in 1891 and 1894 regarding cocaine in medical practice. Most respondents felt a "great responsibility" when prescribing cocaine. The most common method of dealing with this concern was simply to hide the identity of the drug from the patient.[54]

Perhaps inevitably, the call for self-regulation meshed with the growing concern over the numbers of poorly educated physicians. In other words, blame for the overuse of cocaine might lie with doctors seeking to compensate for lack of ability through potent drugging with morphine and cocaine. One such critic, Heine Marks, complained that "a host of these incompetents is turned loose every year, and their ranks are being constantly augmented." Marks regarded these physicians with contempt and as a sign that "there are too many medical colleges in this country." As for their use of cocaine, "too often they tell their patients what they are giving to relieve them . . . I am not one who believes that a physician should thus take his patients into his confidence. There are entirely too many of that sort of pseudo-partnerships."[55]

The individual-idiosyncrasy theory of the cocaine habit buoyed hopes for self-regulation. Of course, the nature of the theory varied: a physical or chemical imbalance, nervousness and other psychological explanations, family history, or racial and ethnic background. Both defenders and critics of cocaine employed the idiosyncrasy theory. Advocates such as Freud and Hammond came up with their own idiosyncrasy theory to explain the incidence of cocaine abuse: only individuals with a prior history of drug or alcohol abuse became cocaine abusers.[56] H. G. Brainerd of Los Angeles, analyzing six cases of the cocaine habit, described the general logic of the idiosyncrasy theory. The lethal dose of cocaine varied from person to person so that a deadly dose for one patient might be taken "without serious results" by another. Thus, argued Brainerd, one could explain why some patients apparently avoided a habit, even after long periods of use, whereas others seemed hooked "almost from the first dose."[57] Identifying susceptible persons could pave the way for continued use of cocaine by "normal" people.[58]

Finally, the demographics of users and habitués helped shape the more optimistic view that the cocaine habit was more of a problematic by-product of therapeutic practice than a danger to public safety. The transformation of the opiate addict from the middle-aged, female opium addict of the 1870s to the young, male heroin addict of the 1920s precipitated a shift toward medical and public condemnation of addicts.[59] By the late nineteenth century, physicians had already divided opiate addicts into those whose addiction derived from the therapeutic use of opium or morphine and those who were the so-called "pleasure users." Similarly, both medical and popular opinions were considerably less aroused by cocaine habitués in the era of medical use than by subsequent generations of cocaine consumers.

An examination of twenty-eight case histories reported in the medical literature strongly suggests that a typical cocaine addict in the 1880s and 1890s was a male professional in his early thirties who had begun using cocaine in the treatment of a medical complaint. Of the twenty-eight cases, twenty-seven were men. Although the patient's age was given in only ten instances, the average age was just under thirty-three years. Most of these addicts (seventeen of twenty-eight) were also physicians. Another eight were professionals of some sort, and no profession was listed for the remaining three cases. T. D. Crothers, in an 1898 article for the *Quarterly Journal of Inebriety,* drew the profile in the same terms: "The cocaine-takers are usually past 30, and most of them have taken alcohol or opium and other drugs for their effects before cocaine was used. A much larger proportion of professional men are victims in proportion to other classes."[60]

That physicians constituted the largest group of cocaine habitués in the medical era is certain. As late as 1898, physicians were thought to constitute 30 percent of those with the habit. This pattern was not unusual because physicians had also been among the leading abusers of morphine and chloral hydrate. So familiar was the profession's propensity to overuse new drugs that even physicians inclined to discount the extent of cocaine abuse warned their colleagues against self-prescription. E. W. Holmes concluded an otherwise positive article on the therapeutic use of cocaine with a warning to colleagues in the form of the old adage, "A man his own lawyer has a fool for his client."[61] Nearly every general commentary on the cocaine habit mentioned its prevalence among physicians.[62]

The prevalence of self-experimentation among physicians probably explains the high incidence of the cocaine habit. The absence of any formal process by which drug experimentation took place in the nineteenth century encouraged physicians to experiment on themselves in an effort to devise applications for new drug products,[63] simply "to see what effect it would produce."[64] The unfortunate story of William Halsted and his research assistants illustrates the point well. Halsted and others injected themselves with cocaine repeatedly during their research on the drug's anesthetic effects. Unknown to most, Halsted and several others became cocaine abusers. The symptoms of his abuse caused such concern among his colleagues that his friend William Henry Welch hired a schooner and sailed with Halsted to the Windward Islands in an attempt to separate him from cocaine. Halsted ultimately "cured" himself of his cocaine abuse by adopting morphine use instead, no less of a habit, but one that allowed him to proceed with one of the most notable careers in American surgery. His three cocaine-abusing fellow researchers died without abandoning their use of cocaine.[65]

In addition to the propensity in the medical community for abusing new drugs, the very nature of the therapeutic application of cocaine recommended it to professionals. Cocaine use in overcoming mental exhaustion and overwork seemed to confine it to patients of a more refined temperament and the so-called brain workers. Although its use was never entirely restricted to such "elites," there is evidence that most early addicts were professional men. In a report to the *Quarterly Journal of Inebriety,* T. D. Crothers gave several examples of cocaine-induced behavior. Although these examples primarily depict the cocaine addict's appearance, they also reinforce the demographic profile presented earlier of the typical cocaine addict in the 1880s and 1890s. Crothers included in his report the following: "a club man of wealth and prominence, known to drink wine at the table, and occasionally to excess, became deliriously exhilarated, boasting of his strength of both body and mind"; "a noted lawyer became very diffusive in his conversation and pleas to the jury, going on without point or conclusion, almost indefinitely"; "a teacher of medicine will occasionally lose all sense of proportion in his lectures and spend the hour on some insignificant part of the subject, or digress to another topic, never realizing this change."[66] Such persons — "victims" of cocaine — aroused sympathy rather scorn from their peers.

The therapeutically addicted professional avoided the punitive treatment of the so-called social drug taker. In the 1880s and 1890s, the most notable of these were opium smokers, whose habit was considered a vice and a gratification of abnormal desires. Heine Marks, in calling for more sensible use of cocaine, referred to opium smoking as the "immoral phase" of opiate use. Marks explicitly linked use and user when he observed that "the immorality of the practice will be conceded when we reflect that most of its devotees there [in the West] are gamblers and prostitutes."[67] If the users were disreputable, so were the opium dens that drew users of all classes, dragging them all down to the same degraded level. As a vice, opium smoking drew a hostile response, whereas the thousands of therapeutically addicted opiate users remained safely classified as "victims" of the habit. These same issues applied to cocaine. Nearly all medical-era habitual users were treated sympathetically as victims, whereas the twentieth century saw the rise of the unsympathetic and punitive term, *cocaine fiend.*[68]

All of the elements of the medical response to the use and abuse of cocaine during these early years come together in the case of Dr. Charles D. Bradley of Chicago, whose experience with the cocaine habit was particularly well documented. Dr. Bradley had begun experimenting with cocaine in May 1885, "having been led to believe it to be a harmless stimulant, and being at the time much run down by excessive professional work." According to D. R. Brower, who was one of Bradley's friends, cocaine "gave him [Bradley] such a sense of well-being as he had never experienced before, the sense of complete repose and self-satisfaction it produced being much more marked than that derived from opium."[69] Bradley increased his dosage until he reached a level of 1 gram per day, injected hypodermically. According to a newspaper account, after taking cocaine for some time, Dr. Bradley's behavior had become increasingly uncontrollable. He used cocaine himself and gave it to members of his family, declaring that he would "revolutionize medicine generally, and become the world's benefactor."[70]

Brower recalled that his friend "was formerly a modest man of science; he became bold and unscientific in his methods . . . threatening vengeance upon all who dared doubt the correctness of his statements, a perfect terror in his neighborhood."[71] In pursuit of cocaine, Bradley mortgaged his home and reduced his family to poverty. Bradley's physical decline paralleled his mental decline; he seldom slept and appeared emaciated and pale. It was then, in November 1885, that Drs. Brower and F. L. Wadsworth brought Bradley to the judge and suggested that he be committed to the Washingtonian Home in the hope of ending his cocaine use. For all his wild behavior, published newspaper accounts were still quite sympathetic to Bradley, referring to him as the "cocaine victim."

Dr. Brower later presented the case to the Chicago Medical Society, where he highlighted a number of effective therapeutic uses of cocaine but also condemned its use in treating inebriety. Brower also concluded that long-term use caused "a very marked deterioration of the central nervous system, producing a profound cerebral neurasthenia, and may produce such a mal-nutrition of the cerebrum as to develop insanity." Such, he felt, was the case with Dr. Bradley. Brower's comments met with considerable response from the assembled physicians, most of whom suggested that the case was exceptional and preventable. Others raised the issue of personal idiosyncrasy, arguing that "it would hardly be reasonable to charge it all to cocaine." In response, Brower generally agreed, conceding that "he did not suppose that such disastrous results" would occur "unless there was some weakness of the nervous system."[72]

As for Dr. Bradley, his stay at the Washingtonian Home was an unsuccessful one. Although his use of cocaine was halted temporarily, he continued to behave erratically. While at the Home, he declared that he was "greatly provoked" by the physicians who thought him insane. Bradley concluded that he had perhaps taken his experiment too far.[73] Shortly afterward, he left the Home for Canada and cocaine. In January 1887, police arrested Bradley in Chicago after he turned on a gas jet at a drugstore where he had been denied cocaine. According to the newspaper account, Bradley was "suffering from acute mania, convulsions, and every distressing phase of violent insanity . . . reduced to a skeleton, and has been practicing every form of deception to procure the drug that has been the cause of his ruin. He will probably be put under permanent restraint this time."[74]

The case of the unfortunate Dr. Bradley suggests the contradictory impulses of the medical profession in responding to cocaine abuse. No one denied that the compulsive use of cocaine had ruined Bradley's medical career, torn apart his family, destroyed his health, and reduced the doctor to living on the street. On the other hand, the profession's response to both cocaine abuse and cocaine poisoning was mitigated by a sense that cocaine was a valuable medical tool if employed conservatively. The costs of cocaine use could be limited through informal controls on the medical use of the drug. Demands for formal regulation of cocaine use and distribution, which would soon be characteristic of the public response of organized medicine to cocaine abuse, played little part in nineteenth-century medical opinion.

The rather subdued medical response to the perceived dangers of cocaine in the era of medical use came from a conviction that physicians could retain their near-exclusive control over use and distribution. Conversely, the instances in which patients continued the use of cocaine independently seemed to hold the greatest potential for trouble. As its medical use became prevalent, physicians indulged the hope that they could retain the "secret" of cocaine. Physicians' greatest fears, however, were about to be realized, as the drug industry destroyed the illusion of medical control and prompted a new generation of physicians to seek ways to establish more formal regulatory authority over all drugs.

THREE

Making Cocaine

The evident excitement in medical circles over the potential new therapeutic uses of cocaine in autumn 1884 drew a rapid response from the drug industry. Many drug trade publications reported the news of Carl Koller's breakthrough within a month of the New York medical journal reports of it. The *American Druggist* noted editorially that "there is reason to believe that this discovery will prove to be one of the greatest importance."[1] The *Oil, Paint, and Drug Reporter,* a New York trade publication, shared the enthusiasm for cocaine but cautioned that the drug industry lacked the capacity to supply the initial demand. The expected increase in consumption, the editors predicted, "will require the exercise of unusual energy to supply the new outlet."[2]

In autumn 1884, the American and European drug industries had almost no capacity to produce cocaine. Coca leaves, the necessary raw material to manufacture cocaine, were scarce in Western marketplaces. What supplies of leaves did turn up in foreign ports were often of very poor quality, having lost part or all of their alkaloid content during transportation. Even if an adequate supply of coca leaves had been available, very few manufacturers had any prior experience with manufacturing cocaine. The few American drug firms that carried small stocks imported the drug from Germany, where the chemical firm of E. Merck & Company manufactured cocaine for distribution by the milligram to researchers.[3] Parke, Davis & Company, the Detroit-based drug firm, had a small stock of Merck's cocaine which they carried for experimental use. Physicians and druggists searching for supplies would normally have looked to drug wholesalers, but before 1884, most of these firms did not carry cocaine. Only the New York firms of McKesson & Robbins and Schieffelin & Company, two of the nation's largest wholesalers, listed cocaine in their catalogs.[4]

Consequently, in late 1884 when physicians sought to obtain cocaine for use or experimentation, they found the supply low and the cost nearly prohibitive.

High prices in Europe nearly prevented Sigmund Freud from beginning his research because the young neurologist was unable to afford cocaine from Merck.[5] The standard price for cocaine in 1884 was $1 per grain or more than $400 per ounce, although it appears that supplies were so low that the sale of an entire ounce would have been improbable. McKesson & Robbins took its small supply of cocaine and sold it as a "special favor" to a few New York physicians and surgeons, "a few grains at a time" at the cost of $1 per grain. The German chemical firm of Gehe & Company reported that "stocks which would have otherwise been sufficient for years were exhausted in a few days. The value of coca leaves very soon advanced until exorbitant prices were charged."[6] Even after significant price reductions in spring 1885, the first whole ounce of cocaine to arrive in the city of Cincinnati cost the retail firm of Martin & Heister $125, a substantial sum for one retail outlet to invest.[7]

Despite the high prices, physicians and drug industry observers who commented on the future of cocaine believed that the demand for it would continue to expand. In 1884, the *Pharmaceutical Record* acknowledged cocaine to be more expensive than "any other known substance used in medicine," yet "so beneficial are the results obtained from a very small amount of it that it is comparatively cheap."[8] Reinforcing industry optimism, a well-known New York surgeon claimed that because surgical applications of cocaine required only small doses of 2 or 4 percent cocaine solution, the price was actually comparable to that of the larger required doses of ether.[9]

Had the drug industry merely been content with supplying the rather limited requirements of surgeons, of course, the underdeveloped state of the cocaine business might have proven satisfactory. Instead, the capacity of the drug industry to manufacture expanded consistently over the next several decades, making cocaine one of the most important products of the European and American pharmaceutical/chemical industry by the turn of the century. Cocaine manufacturers developed a cheap and consistent supply, both affordable and accessible to the American consumer, paving the way for a dramatic increase in the prevalence of cocaine consumption.

The Cocaine Business at the Source of Supply

While physicians scrambled to find reliable supplies of cocaine in November 1884, Henry Hurd Rusby was otherwise occupied developing the botanical collections of Parke, Davis & Company. As a medical student, Rusby had made repeated trips to the American Southwest, collecting botanical specimens for the Smithsonian Institution. Upon his graduation in 1884, Rusby entered the employ of Parke, Davis as the company's botanist, continuing to focus on the plant life of the Southwest.

It must have come as some surprise then, when general manager George S. Davis and chemist Albert B. Lyons approached him that November asking him how soon he could get ready to travel to Bolivia. In his autobiography, Rusby recalled that Davis told him that "there were important commercial possibilities in the then little-known drug coca or Erythroxylon." Although "the use of the leaf as a masticatory by the natives of the Andes had been known since America was discovered," Davis told Rusby, "only a short time before it had been accidentally discovered that a solution of its alkaloid, cocaine, would wholly destroy the local power of sensation in an eye, on coming in contact with the eyeball." Davis and Lyons had determined to study the potential of the new drug, but that "with the exception of small experimental lots, which had been kept for a long time, no supply of the coca leaf existed here."[10] At their urging, Rusby set off to locate sources of the coca leaf in Bolivia and to learn more about this potentially valuable plant (Figure 3.1).[11]

Rusby began his journey without even the most basic information about coca, a problem shared by other interested parties, including the U.S. government. In January 1885, the secretary of the navy wrote to the consulates in Peru and Bolivia, communicating the difficulty in supplying the American market with coca and requesting information concerning "how this product can be brought within reach of the American purchaser."[12]

In his reply, Bolivian Consul-General Richard Gibbs reported what Rusby and others would soon find: the existence of a well-developed coca trade in that country. Gibbs noted that Bolivia recorded and taxed production of about 7.5 million pounds annually. Of this amount, about 55 percent was consumed in Bolivia, with 15 percent going to Argentina, 15 percent to Chile, 10 percent to Peru, and 5 percent to the United States and Europe.[13] Peru and Bolivia produced nearly all of the available coca. Estimates of coca production in these two countries in the early 1880s placed the total between 20 million and 30 million pounds of leaves. Already accustomed to the export trade, Peruvian and Bolivian growers adapted quickly to new demands for American and European exports by increasing production using existing methods of processing and transportation.

The coca-growing regions of South America produced a confusing variety of coca plants, each with some distinctive characteristics (although many were hard to distinguish). Out of Rusby's travels in the service of science and Parke, Davis emerged the idea among manufacturers that these different types of coca might have differing levels of utility. Rusby identified two basic types of coca, a dichotomy that was to guide cocaine manufacturers in the United States. Rusby

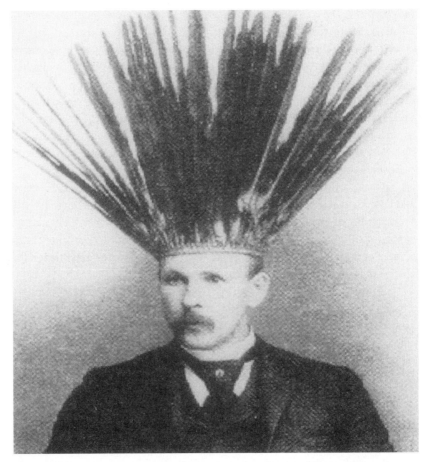

Figure 3.1. Henry Hurd Rusby, botanist and adventurer. In 1885, Henry Hurd Rusby was sent by Parke, Davis to locate a reliable source of coca. Here he appears in native headgear in a photograph originally published in his memoirs, *Jungle Memories.* Courtesy of the Falk Library of the Health Sciences, University of Pittsburgh.

first observed a broad, thick leaf that came to be known in manufacturing circles as the Huanuco leaf. The second type was a narrower, thinner, and more brittle leaf that manufacturers classified as Truxillo coca.[14] Huanuco leaves had a higher cocaine content, but Rusby and others noted that the Truxillo leaf appeared to be the most highly prized by Bolivian and Peruvian coca chewers.[15] As a consequence of this observation, Truxillo leaves found favor with manufacturers of coca products.[16]

Cocaine manufacturers in the United States and Europe rarely pursued ownership of coca plantations, obtaining their coca from independent growers on small farms and large plantations. Workers (sometimes paid with coca) gathered the leaves, which were then laid out and dried by other workers. Once dried, the coca was gathered in 150-pound bales and taken by mules and llamas to regional centers, where the leaves would be purchased by coca dealers.

The transportation of leaves was difficult and time consuming because each mule carried only two bales of leaves over difficult terrain. Although some areas eventually made use of railroads (and some use of rivers, such as the Huallaga in Peru), mule transport remained a vital part of coca production. For export, the leaves were taken to Pacific ports (from north to south: Guayaquil, Salvaverry, Callao, Mollendo, and Arica). There, the leaves were bundled and sealed with turpentine to prevent water and moisture from rotting them, thus avoiding the worst of the earlier problems with spoilage.[17] From these Pacific ports, coca was transported to the isthmus of Panama (then part of Colombia) where it would be taken to the Atlantic terminus of the trans-Panama railroad, Colon. From Colon, the leaves went to ports in Europe and the United States.

Although obtaining supplies of coca at the source was not difficult, the transportation route left manufacturers open to problems of two kinds. First, shipping coca took a considerable amount of time even when transporters encountered no extraordinary problems. Because coca was a product particularly vulnerable to damage and lost alkaloid content with the passage of time, getting the leaves to manufacturers quickly was essential. Efforts to reduce the transportation time from Latin America seem to have met with little success. Edward R. Squibb attempted to make use of the Amazon River, but the experiment failed, and almost no coca ever went to Atlantic ports. Instead, manufacturers seem to have conceded the loss of some cocaine content.[18]

In addition, suppliers rarely enjoyed optimal transportation conditions for any length of time. Everything from a llama shortage to a cholera epidemic periodically reduced coca exports to a trickle.[19] The many conflicts and insurrections in Peru, Bolivia, and Colombia caused the most serious disruptions in supply. In 1886, the *American Druggist* reported that "the numerous revolutions and constant wars, without which Peru and Bolivia do not seem to be able to exist, have been a serious obstacle to the development of the industry."[20] A decade later, the *Oil, Paint, and Drug Reporter* observed that "little disturbances, generally called rebellions, are apt to occur at almost any time in the republics lying to the south of us, and they usually come without much warning to the outside world."[21] An insurrection in Colombia diverted Rusby's entire initial shipment of leaves to Parke, Davis, and Peruvian unrest in 1894–95 and 1900 resulted in temporary cessation of coca exports.

Growing demand for cocaine in the United States resulted in a significant expansion of coca cultivation in Peru and Bolivia. In 1885, E. R. Squibb had estimated that Peru harvested 15 million pounds of leaves annually and Bolivia 7.5 million. Louis Lewin, writing in the early 1920s, estimated the size of Peruvian and Bolivian crops at 33 million and 17.5 million pounds, respectively.[22]

Much of the expansion in Peru took place in the north of the country, where coca had traditionally been less important as a crop than in the area around Cuzco. Before the 1880s, the coca grown in this district had supplied regional demand, mostly from mine workers. By the late 1890s, the district coca fields supplied nearly 200,000 pounds of leaves and expanded in the first decade of the twentieth century to more than 400,000 pounds of coca annually. Similar expansions of coca planting took place in other regions of Peru as well as in Bolivia. A report in the *American Druggist* noted that coca cultivation was no longer "limited to the localities most favored by the climate and the low price of labor."[23]

Manufacturing interests also looked to cultivate coca outside the traditional exporting nations. Manufacturers hoped to reduce the time and cost of transportation from South America. Firms in the United States, for example, engaged in a futile search for domestic growing sites for coca.[24] European colonial powers sought to produce valuable coca in their own territories, thus securing a more advantageous position in the global cocaine market. Growers marveled at the ease with which coca could be introduced into suitable climates. As one scholar concluded recently, "coca must be the world's easiest cash crop to cultivate."[25] A report from British India on the potential for coca cultivation enthused, "it grows like a weed."[26]

Some of the earliest attempts to expand cultivation outside traditional areas took place where some variety of the coca plant already grew. In Colombia, the Magdelena River valley continued to supply the large number of native coca users. A 1912 expedition reported extensive production in the region around Cali, Colombia, "in the door-yard of almost every house."[27] Varieties also grew in Brazil, where systematic cultivation appears to have failed to produce a substantial crop for export.

A report published in the *British and Colonial Druggist* noted that "this Erythroxylon is easily grown, and might well be introduced upon a commercial scale in Australia, India, and other British colonies, with manifold advantages, both pharmaceutical and financial." The report even suggested that coca cultivation might succeed in Britain; the author had kept some coca plants alive through the winter in Devonshire.[28] A limited success was achieved in British India, where coca production began in 1894 in the Nilgiris region. Because of competition from cheap South American coca, however, most of this coca was consumed domestically.[29] British planters in Ceylon, discontented with low prices for their cinchona bark, took up the cultivation of coca in the late 1880s. None of the Ceylon coca reached American manufacturers in anything other than experimental lots, although growers eventually exported their product to British manufacturers.[30] By 1914, nearly all of the coca imported into Britain was grown in Ceylon. In both Ceylon and India the type of coca introduced was *Erythroxylon novogranatense*, sometimes referred to as Colombian coca.

By far the most successful alternative growing venture outside Latin America before 1920 was in the Dutch East Indies on the island of Java.[31] Already a major production center for opium, Javanese growers apparently began cultivating *Erythroxylon novogranatense* in the late 1880s in the area around Batavia (now Jakarta).[32] Until the twentieth century, the amount of coca leaves was very limited, with only about 500 acres under cultivation. A report from the island in 1908 suggested that there was "room for considerable extension" of the worldwide cocaine market and that Javanese coca might be its source. Once planted, coca produced a quick return, making it an ideal crop for new rubber plantations because rubber crops took more time to develop. A planting of coca might produce a valuable crop in as little as one year.

After 1900, growers in Java shipped the leaves to the Nederlandsche Cocainefabriek [hereafter NCF] in Amsterdam as well as the Cheiron factory in Bussum and the Brocades and Steehman factory in Meppel, helping the Dutch to become the third largest manufacturer of cocaine after Germany and the United States. Table 3.1 suggests the extent of the growth in Javanese coca exports.

Javanese coca growers and Dutch cocaine manufacturers capitalized on the disruptions caused by World War I to increase their share of the world market. The traditional supply routes of cocaine to the United States from Germany and of coca leaves from South America were reduced greatly and replaced largely by Java coca and Dutch cocaine (Table 3.2).

TABLE 3.1
Coca Exports, Java

Year	Amount (in Metric Tons)
1891	16
1904	26
1911	740
1912	800
1920	1,700

SOURCES: 1891: *Oil, Paint, and Drug Reporter;* 1904, 1911, 1912, 1920: Louis Lewin, *Phantastica: Narcotic and Stimulating Drugs, Their Use and Abuses* (1931; reprint, New York: E. P. Dutton, 1964), 78.

TABLE 3.2
Coca from Port of Origin (New York Arrivals)

Source	1912	1916
Panama	437,988	97,395
Netherlands	47,620	158,125
Java	0	258,750
Germany	22,315	0
Peru	22,212	0
Other	2,034	23,850

SOURCE: *Oil, Paint, and Drug Reporter* weekly importation reports.

According to *Merck's Report* in 1917, Java coca planters "seem about to crowd the South American coca leaves more and more from the market." Eventually, resentment over the loss of part of the coca market led to a measure prohibiting the export of viable coca seeds from Bolivia.[33]

Coca cultivation expanded with striking ease in both new and traditional regions. The Java experience demonstrates the capacity of growers in one region to accommodate demand caused by disruptions in other areas. In the case of Java, although World War I cut off American supplies of German cocaine and made South American coca harder to obtain, manufacturers in the United States found a ready alternative source. Over time, the business of coca cultivation revealed a considerable capacity to expand and sustain itself.

Crude Cocaine Production and Falling Prices

Establishing the manufacture of crude cocaine at plants close to the source of the supply of coca leaves proved to be the most significant development in the production of cocaine, contributing to dramatic price decreases after 1884. The manufacture of crude cocaine involved the processing of leaves to extract the cocaine alkaloid, which was then exported to foreign markets for the final stages of extraction. Cocaine producers had several reasons to favor such a system of production. First, processing the leaves in South American plants allowed the alkaloids to be extracted from coca leaves while the leaves were still fresh and green and generated a slightly higher yield of cocaine. Second, crude cocaine did not suffer during transportation, arriving in the condition in which it was shipped. Third, the high cost of transporting bulky coca leaves could be reduced by shipping the much more compact cargoes of crude cocaine. Fourth, the production of crude cocaine required little capital investment or skilled industrial labor, neither of which was in great supply in the major growing regions.

Various drug industry representatives proposed to process coca leaves closer to the source almost immediately after Koller's experiments. In a February 1885 editorial, the *National Druggist* highlighted the ways in which the manufacture of crude cocaine in South America could reduce manufacturers' costs (and those of consumers as well), concluding that "if there was ever an argument in favor of manufacturing an article of this kind in its native country, such an argument is supplied in the case of coca."[34] When Parke, Davis sent Rusby to South America in search of a supply of coca, the firm also equipped the botanist with a distilling apparatus. George S. Davis was hopeful that Rusby might produce some cocaine where he found the leaves. The process by which Rusby was to manufacture the cocaine was experimental, however, and the first shipment to Parke, Davis turned out to be unusable. Rusby and Parke, Davis got no second chance because the distilling equipment blew up shortly afterward.[35]

Despite this false start, crude cocaine manufacture in South America made rapid advances. Peruvian sources suggest that at least two Lima firms were offering crude cocaine as early as 1885 and may have begun experimental production even earlier. The first European company to establish crude cocaine production was the chemical firm of Boehringer & Soehne of Mannheim, Germany. Boehringer & Soehne sent a chemist to Lima, Peru, in late 1884 to set up a production facility, which began full operations in 1885.[36] A French pharmaceutical journal described the process of manufacturing crude cocaine:

> The leaves are mashed with a concentrated solution of sodium carbonate. The mixture is evaporated in the sun, and the powder is exhausted with benzin or petroleum-ether, and is shaken with a solution of hydrochloric acid. Precipitation with sodium carbonate then liberates the crude cocaine, which is purified in Europe or the United States.[37]

The "crude" cocaine that left South America was about 80 to 90 percent pure in the first several years of production, reported to be 95 percent pure in the mid 1890s, and as much as 98.5 to 99 percent pure in 1904.

Although Boehringer established its own crude cocaine factory, most companies that manufactured cocaine did not control this aspect of the process. Instead, they relied on independent growers and independent processing facilities to supply the intermediate material for their finished products.[38] These independent operators could occasionally disrupt the cocaine business, as when Peruvian crude cocaine factories shut down after disagreements with customs authorities. Few cocaine manufacturers ever integrated all levels of the production process into their South American operations, relying on independent coca growers and crude processing facilities.

Although most cocaine manufacturers did not control the production of crude cocaine, for persons with the resources to set up a simple factory and access to the proper chemicals, the crude cocaine business was an attractive enterprise. According to a report from Peru in the late 1890s, 100 kilograms of coca leaves cost the crude cocaine manufacturer between 15 and 20 soles but could produce approximately 180 soles worth of cocaine. Within two years, four factories were producing crude cocaine. A decade later, ten factories in Peru were processing it. Five were located in Huanuco, two in Lima, one in Callao, one in the Menon district, and one in the Puzuzo district. In 1901 and 1905, Peru reported the operation of twenty-one crude cocaine factories.[39] Coca growers seeking to expand their trade owned some of these factories. European chemical companies had direct ownership and operation of a few, although this was relatively uncommon. Foreign-born Peruvians (especially Germans and Japanese) with no direct connection to chemical or pharmaceutical firms owned the remainder.

In Peru, the amount of coca leaves consumed in crude cocaine manufacture eventually came to exceed the amount of unprocessed leaves exported. A report from the German consulate at Callao indicated that production in 1901 was dominated by crude cocaine manufacture. That year, Peru manufactured and exported more than 10,700 kilograms of cocaine (the all-time peak of production), which corresponded to the use of more than 1,500 tons of coca leaves. The export of coca leaves from Peru the same year totaled 610 tons. The same report noted that the production of cocaine in 1901 was double that of 1897, highlighting a remarkable period of growth in the Peruvian crude cocaine business.[40]

The importation of crude cocaine affected the European cocaine industry most of all. The German chemical industry, the largest and most advanced in Europe, embraced the idea of using crude cocaine in the manufacture of the pure product. Imports of crude cocaine rapidly replaced coca leaves as the source of most German-manufactured cocaine. Table 3.3 shows the importation of crude cocaine and coca leaves into Hamburg, the center of Germany's cocaine manufacturing and "the principal crude cocaine market of the world."

Although the importation of coca fluctuated over the years, the importation of crude cocaine experienced consistent growth, nearly fourfold from 1892 through 1904. All available sources suggest that German production continued to rise after 1904. A 1923 report indicated that by the start of the war in 1914, German cocaine production approached 20,000 kilograms.[41]

German manufacturers established the first crude cocaine plants, but American and Dutch manufacturers continued to rely primarily on cocaine produced domestically from imported coca leaves. One factor in the continuing importance

TABLE 3.3
*Crude Cocaine Imports and Manufactured Cocaine
from Coca Leaf Imports, Hamburg (in Kilograms)*

Year	Imported Crude	Cocaine from Coca (Estimated)
1881		10
1886		430
1887		155
1890		890
1891		225
1892	1,735	645
1893		530
1894	2,382	450
1895		530
1897	2,407	360
1898		345
1899	3,280	660
1900	4,210	565
1901	4,595	
1902	5,817	567
1903	5,642	
1904	6,443	

SOURCE: *Handels-Bericht von Gehe & Company* published annual reports from the collections of the American Institute of the History of Pharmacy, Gehe & Company file, Kremers Reference Files.

of coca leaves to American manufacturers was the shorter transportation time involved relative to German manufacturers. The most critical factor in the decision by American manufacturers to employ coca leaves was an *ad valorem* duty of 25 percent on imported crude cocaine. Because coca leaves could be imported duty free, using crude cocaine was not an attractive option for American firms.[42] For reasons that are not entirely clear, the Philadelphia chemical firm of Powers-Weightman-Rosengarten proved to be an exception to this general rule, relying exclusively on crude cocaine manufactured in Peru.[43]

Although manufacturers in the United States and elsewhere continued to use imported coca leaves in their manufacture of cocaine, the development of crude cocaine production affected markets well beyond Germany. Most notably, the business in crude cocaine reduced further the cost of manufactured cocaine in Germany, reductions that other international manufacturers had to match. The price of cocaine dropped precipitously from approximately $1 per grain in 1884–85 to 2¢ per grain by 1887.[44]

The expansion and improvement of cocaine manufacturing after 1885 helped to change cocaine from a rare and expensive drug to a common and inexpensive one. In fact, the catalog price of an ounce of cocaine during 1885 depended largely on how early in the year the price was quoted. In Pittsburgh, wholesale firms quoted the price of cocaine at $1 per grain in January. The Parke, Davis price list issued early in the year showed cocaine at $280 per ounce. Later in the year, the Chicago per ounce price of cocaine fell to $150, and the price quoted by Schieffelin at $130 per ounce was the lowest on the market. By September, the Chicago price had fallen to 10¢ per grain, or just over $40 per ounce.[45] Prices fell through much of the next decade (see Figure 3.2). On two subsequent occasions, prices rose and then declined again. The first increase, around 1900, resulted from disruptions at the source of supply. As Figure 3.2 indicates, the price began to decline again in late 1901, reaching bottom in July 1908 at its all-time lowest wholesale per-ounce price of $2. The second rise began late in 1908 because of an increase in the import duty. Although this increase was more gradual than the earlier rise in price, manufacturers again appear to have responded by gradually reducing the price to about $3 per ounce by 1914. (The final increase shown was a result of the beginning of the war in Europe.) The price of coca leaves also experienced a marked decline after 1885. Figure 3.2 shows the long-term trends in the price of coca; a comparison of cocaine and coca prices from 1892 through 1916 shows the close link between the two products.

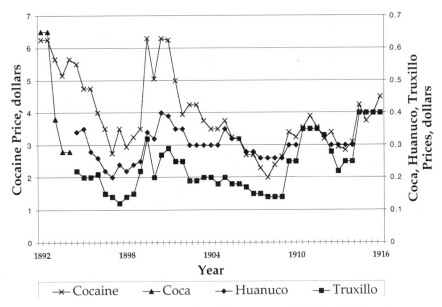

Figure 3.2. Wholesale prices of coca and cocaine, 1892–1916. Weekly wholesale price reports, *Oil, Paint, and Drug Reporter.*

The Cocaine Manufacturers

European and American companies controlled the manufacture of pure cocaine. Although pharmaceutical firms (those that manufactured drug products
for medical use) were the first to enter the business, chemical manufacturers became the largest presence. Chemical manufacturers specialized in the large-scale
production of specific medicinal chemicals such as chloral hydrate, morphine,
and quinine. By contrast, pharmaceutical manufacturers prepared mainly dosage
level products and drug compounds. In Germany, where a strong chemical industry developed earlier, such firms (including Merck, Gehe, Boehringer, Zimmer, and others) dominated the production of pure cocaine.

Given the underdevelopment of the U.S. chemical industry in the late nineteenth century, the critical steps toward cocaine production involved pharmaceutical companies. Three firms contributed the most: E. R. Squibb & Company,
McKesson & Robbins, and Parke, Davis. Edward R. Squibb's company was
among the most influential pharmaceutical manufacturers, not because of its size
(Squibb did not develop sales of significant size until after Squibb's two sons sold
the firm in 1905) but because of the enormous influence that Edward Squibb held
over the practice of pharmacy and drug development. Even as Squibb's criticisms
of coca before 1884 helped deflate the demand for coca, his enthusiastic reversal
after Koller's discoveries paved the way for extensive cocaine manufacture.

Squibb's most extensive involvement with cocaine came early. He began to
manufacture cocaine in October 1884, the same month in which Koller's experiments were first reported. At first, Squibb was only able to produce "a few grains"
of crystal cocaine and a few ounces of cocaine in solution for his customers, but
he rapidly began importing coca leaves for further production. According to
Squibb, the company actually lost money on many of these early transactions because of the high cost of developing new production processes. From October
1884 through October 1886, Squibb purchased 22,285 pounds of coca leaves.
Given coca importation figures, this probably represented about 5 percent of the
total coca consumption in the United States (Squibb also employed additional
coca leaves in the manufacture of coca products).[46] Squibb's personal interest,
however, was the development and application of new drug products. As cocaine
became an established drug, efficiently manufactured by the chemical industry,
Squibb stopped pursuing cocaine sales.

Before 1884 the New York firm of McKesson & Robbins was among the leading importers of coca and one of the few companies that offered small amounts
of cocaine to its customers in that period. Although McKesson & Robbins was
primarily a wholesale drug company, it also imported and manufactured some

drug products, including cocaine. The company claimed to be the first and largest cocaine manufacturer in the United States, making all of its product from coca leaves imported into New York. Coca importation data from the late 1880s confirm that McKesson imported between 20 and 30 percent of all leaves entering New York each year, usually the largest proportion of any single manufacturer. The families who controlled McKesson & Robbins also owned the New York Quinine and Chemical Works, which gradually took over the cocaine business from McKesson.[47]

The most active cocaine manufacturer and promoter in the 1880s and early 1890s was Parke, Davis & Company. Unlike E. R. Squibb, Parke, Davis was in the cocaine-manufacturing business to stay. Through World War I, Parke, Davis was the only American pharmaceutical firm with a significant capacity for cocaine manufacture. The cocaine that the company produced supplied not only its own pharmaceutical sales but also those of patent medicine manufacturers. Near the peak of its production, Parke, Davis manufactured approximately 13,000 ounces of cocaine per year, which, in the early 1890s, would have accounted for about 20 percent of the American market, a share that fell to less than 10 percent by 1910.

As important as Squibb, McKesson & Robbins, and Parke, Davis were to the early development of cocaine manufacture in the United States, most cocaine came from chemical companies.[48] When physicians introduced cocaine in the 1880s, the German chemical industry dominated the world market in medicinal chemicals. Cocaine was no exception; by 1890, imports of German cocaine exceeded domestic production of cocaine from imported coca leaves. The first German leader in cocaine manufacture was E. Merck of Darmstadt. Merck had begun manufacture of cocaine on a limited basis even before 1884. After 1884, Merck responded to the interest in the drug by expanding production to include a substantial export business with the United States. In 1891, Merck established an American branch, known as Merck & Company, and became the first German firm to distribute cocaine bearing its own label.[49] Other important German cocaine manufacturers, such as Gehe & Company, Knoll & Company, I. D. Reidel, and Zimmer & Company, all supplied the American market through import firms such as Lehn & Fink.[50]

The largest producer among all cocaine manufacturers was C. F. Boehringer & Soehne of Mannheim. In an advertising notice in the *Practical Druggist,* Boehringer asked its customers to "insist on the best," claiming its status as "largest makers in the world of cocaine" and a "special leader" in its manufacture. As late as 1908, the firm pressed its claim to be the "largest makers in the world of quinine sulphate and cocaine hydrochlorate."[51] Like most German manufacturers, Boehringer imported crude cocaine for final processing.

Gradually, American and Dutch chemical firms challenged the primacy of German cocaine manufacturers. The four most important were the Philadelphia firm of Powers-Weightman-Rosengarten, the New York Quinine and Chemical Works, Mallinckrodt Chemical Works of St. Louis, and the NCF in Amsterdam.[52] Of these, only Powers-Weightman-Rosengarten employed crude cocaine imported from South America; the rest used coca leaves.[53] In a 1909 advertisement, Mallinckrodt challenged the place of Boehringer as the world's leading manufacturer of cocaine; one year later the NCF also claimed to be the largest single cocaine producer in the world.

These competing claims of superiority suggest a competitive field of manufacturers. The number of chemical firms actively producing cocaine at any one time varied, but there seem to have been between six and eight major manufacturers after the turn of the century, with a larger number of minor firms. No single cocaine maker ever dominated a majority of the market or even produced more than one third of worldwide production.

Cocaine ranked among the most advertised and promoted products of the extensive lines of medical and industrial chemicals (see Figure 3.3).[54] The two most important products were still morphine and quinine; not even cocaine was as financially significant. Of the remaining chemical products, however, the dollar value of cocaine sales probably exceeded that of any other single product, in part because its price remained higher than most, even as sales declined over time. Mallinckrodt records from 1920, for example, show that the company earned higher gross profits ($125,000) from cocaine than from any other single product except morphine ($220,300).[55]

How Much Cocaine? Measuring Legal Production

Clearly, overall cocaine consumption grew during the late nineteenth and early twentieth centuries when the drug was legally available to consumers. However, the precise pattern of growth in cocaine consumption remains uncertain. How quickly did cocaine use increase, and was the increase consistent or variable over time? When did cocaine use begin to decline, and how rapidly? Providing reasonably accurate estimates of trends in cocaine consumption is no simple matter. It is worth pursuing, however, not only because it challenges the historical imagination but also because it lays a basis for assessing the efficacy of regulatory efforts and the assumptions upon which such efforts were based.

There are no comprehensive data bases from which to collect accurate measures of cocaine use around the turn of the century. No consistent data on cocaine manufacture or importation appear to have been kept before the passage of the

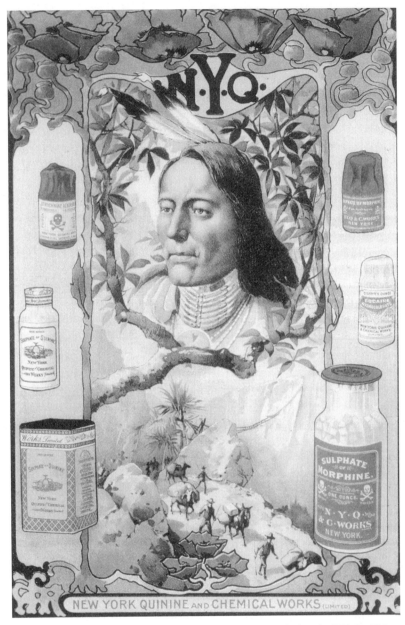

Figure 3.3. 1901 advertisement from the New York Quinine and Chemical Works. This advertisement promotes the most important drug products of the firm: morphine, quinine, and cocaine. The link between the modern drug industry and traditional medicines is represented by the opium poppies and cinchona foliage at the top and the coca gatherers at the center. The North American Indian suggests the connection that the firm wanted to make between their modern products and traditional folk wisdom. Courtesy of the American Institute of the History of Pharmacy.

Harrison Narcotic Act in 1914. No law or regulation required companies importing cocaine, crude cocaine, or coca leaves to report the amount they brought into the United States. The only required reporting was for paying import duties on drugs, and even then the products were reported in aggregate categories such as "medicinal preparations."

Pharmaceutical and chemical companies, moreover, regarded information about their production of cocaine as private. They rarely made public disclosure of their drug production. Anticocaine sentiment that developed by the turn of the century made the prospect of disclosure even less likely. No one was more aware of this secrecy than Hamilton Wright, United States delegate to the International Opium Commission and Conferences. In 1909, Wright attempted to estimate American cocaine production by requesting data from manufacturers. Although Wright wrote with the authority of the United States Department of State, no company offered him any useful information. Most, like Powers-Weightman-Rosengarten, told Wright that "your question . . . puts us in an embarrassing position, as we have always kept this information to ourselves . . . we cannot permit our competitors to become aware of the details of our business, and they are certainly not entitled to the knowledge."[56] Similar requests to wholesale drug firms met with similar evasions. The day after he received an unsatisfactory reply from Powers-Weightman-Rosengarten, Wright received a letter from the Philadelphia-based wholesale drug firm of John Wyeth & Brothers, which informed him that its data would be of no interest and suggested that he request information from its supplier, Powers-Weightman-Rosengarten.[57] Cocaine manufacturer secrecy effectively prevented Wright and others from securing accurate production estimates.

Coca leaf importation records provide the most common data available to scholars seeking to estimate cocaine consumption. However, no consistent measure of nationwide imports covers the entire period from the 1880s to the 1910s. Commerce Department aggregate data began to appear in the late 1890s but do not provide a reliable measure until 1903. The most useful data for the earlier period came from the pages of the trade publication *Oil, Paint, and Drug Reporter,* which did provide accurate weekly import totals for New York City alone, covering arrivals of all products, from aloes to varnish. Listings of coca imports included the name of the importing company, the amount imported (measured in both bales and by weight), the port of origin, and the name of the vessel on which it arrived. Although the journal listings did not always carry all of these items (the importing firm and the weight were occasionally omitted), the number of bales was always reported. A bale of coca generally had a consistent weight, usually between 120 and 135 pounds. It is thus possible to estimate the total weight of unlisted bales by multiplying the number of such bales by the average weight of the listed bales.

The New York import statistics clearly reveal the basic upward trend in coca consumption. Whereas small amounts of coca leaf were imported before 1885, the usefulness of cocaine in medical practice spurred a huge increase in coca imports, from 24,450 pounds in 1884 to 191,568 pounds in 1885 (see Figure 3.4). Even the 1885 figure was quite low compared with the peak years of coca consumption which lay ahead. After years of a general upward trend, coca imports peaked at 1,277,604 pounds in 1905 and remained fairly steady the following year.

What fraction of the national coca imports did the New York data represent? A conservative estimate, based on a comparison of the New York import statistics with Commerce Department data from 1905 forward, suggests that New York received about 50 percent of all imports into the United States. Some historical reports suggest that New York received only one third of total imports. T. D. Crothers, in particular, argued that the value of coca and cocaine imports at

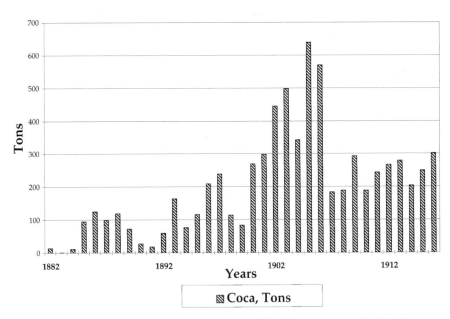

Figure 3.4. New York City coca imports, 1882–1916. Coca imports, reported weekly in the *Oil, Paint, and Drug Reporter,* included both the number of bales and the weight in pounds. Where only the number of bales was reported, the weight was estimated using the average of all other bales that year.

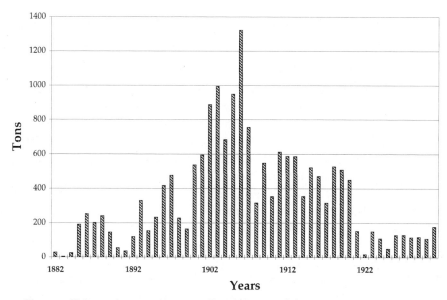

Figure 3.5. U.S. coca imports, 1882–1931. Coca import totals between 1882 and 1904 were calculated as if New York imports represented half of the national total. Import totals after 1904 are based on Commerce Department reports.

New York in 1897 was $150,000 compared with $300,000 at all other ports. The best that can safely be said then is that coca imports through New York represented one third to one half of the entire U.S. consumption. Figure 3.5 joins Commerce Department statistics on U.S. coca imports from 1905 onward with pre-1905 estimates of U.S. imports calculated as if New York imports represented one half the actual total. This is a conservative measure; if, in fact, the New York imports represented only one third of the U.S. total, the pre-1905 estimates would have to be increased substantially.

Having suggested how much coca leaf was imported, how much cocaine does this coca probably represent? Answering this question requires a reliable estimate of how much coca was used in the manufacture of cocaine. Unfortunately, this problem of historical detection has never been addressed satisfactorily. Scholars in both the past and present have derived different estimates of cocaine consumption based on divergent, unstated, and questionable assumptions about how many pounds of coca were required to produce one pound of cocaine.

There appear to be two main schools of thought. In the first is a low estimate, ranging from 100 to 130 pounds of coca necessary to produce a pound of cocaine. A Treasury Department report issued in 1919, for example, suggested that the annual imports of approximately 1 million pounds of coca were sufficient to manufacture 150,000 ounces of cocaine, that is, about 120 pounds of coca per pound of cocaine.[58] This low estimate was repeated in 1975 by Richard Ashley (125 pounds of coca) and by Joel Phillips in 1980 (100–133 pounds of coca).[59] In the second group, the scholars agreed on a higher figure, about 200 pounds of coca per pound of cocaine. Terry and Pellens, writing in the 1920s, used 200 pounds as their benchmark, as did Lawrence Kolb and A. G. DuMez in 1924.[60]

The actual figure, however, lies in between these two estimates. The yield of cocaine alkaloid from reasonably *fresh* Peruvian coca leaves approximates the lower estimate by the Treasury Department in 1919. Results from crude cocaine manufacturing facilities in South America, as contained in a 1901 survey of the crude cocaine business in Peru, appear to support this conclusion. The manufacturing records of the Mallinckrodt company further reinforce this conclusion. Records kept between 1905 and 1909 suggest that an average of about 129 pounds of coca leaves was required to yield one pound of the alkaloid (the averages for the four reporting periods were 123.7, 125.3, 129.5, and 137.8 pounds).

Cocaine manufacturers were never able to "crystallize" all of the cocaine alkaloid, however, making the lower estimates misleading. The Mallinckrodt production records, for example, indicate that the company was able to turn an average of 80.62 percent of the alkaloid into usable cocaine hydrochloride, meaning that 160 pounds of leaf would produce one pound of cocaine hydrochloride. This figure would almost surely have been slightly higher before improvements in the quality of coca leaves, particularly in the 1880s. This figure may also have been somewhat lower as coca leaves from the Dutch East Indies came to dominate the market; Java leaves contained higher percentages of alkaloid, and improvements in manufacturing methods started to produce higher yields.

Using 160 pounds as a best estimate, Figure 3.6 portrays over time the minimum amounts of cocaine which the imported coca leaves would yield. The results indicate that in 1906, at the peak of coca importation, approximately 8.2 tons of cocaine were imported in the form of coca leaves and that an annual average of least 5.9 tons in coca leaves was imported between 1902 and 1906.

Although coca imports provide a good minimum estimate of cocaine consumption, they fail to account for another important factor: imports of crude cocaine and cocaine hydrochloride. Unfortunately, few scholars have taken into account the absence of cocaine imports in estimating turn-of-the-century cocaine consumption in the United States. This is true even for studies done at the time, whose authors should have been aware of cocaine imports.

As the preceding account of cocaine manufacturing suggests, ignoring cocaine importation means seriously underestimating total cocaine consumption.

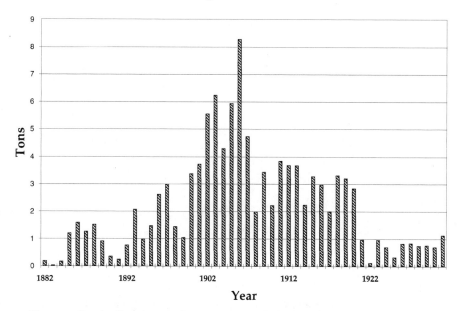

Figure 3.6. Cocaine from imported coca, 1882–1931. Estimates of cocaine produced from imported coca are based upon coca importation in Figure 3.4, with an average yield of 1 pound of cocaine per 160 pounds of leaves.

Furthermore, it may also mean distorting trends in cocaine use because an increase in cocaine imports may well have balanced a corresponding decline in coca imports. At least half of the firms selling cocaine in the United States manufactured the drug outside the country; their sales would be entirely overlooked by coca import data. Other companies, such as Lehn & Fink and C. Bischoff, were importers of German cocaine. Their substantial business would also be ignored by coca import statistics. Finally, one American manufacturer, Powers-Weightman-Rosengarten of Philadelphia, employed crude cocaine from South America in the production of cocaine hydrochloride. Any estimate that relies solely on coca imports ignores the entire production of this company.

Reconstructing turn-of-the-century data on cocaine imports is a task even more challenging than for coca imports because the reporting of cocaine imports was much less reliable. As indicated, pharmaceutical companies were required to report their cocaine only for the purpose of paying the 25 percent duty on the drug. This had several implications for the quality of the data. Manufacturers paying the duty could report the cocaine in its general category, "medicinal preparation"; this aggregate reporting was encouraged by the relatively small size of co-

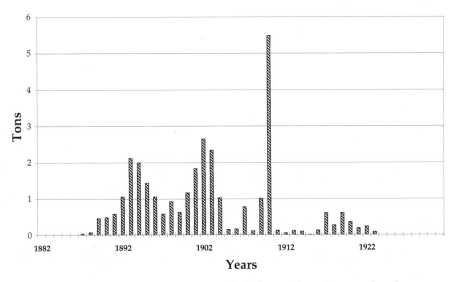

Figure 3.7. U.S. cocaine imports, 1882–1931. Totals for 1882 through 1897 are based on weekly reports in the *Oil, Paint, and Drug Reporter,* estimated to represent half of the national total. Totals from 1898 are based on annual Commerce Department reports.

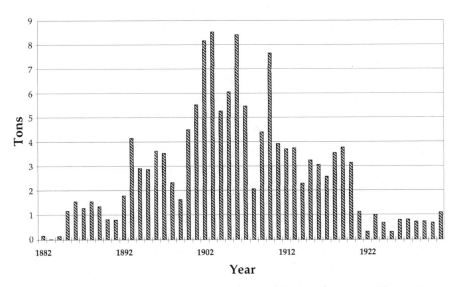

Figure 3.8. Total manufactured and imported cocaine, 1882–1931. Estimates of the total legal cocaine supply are derived from the sum of the import data represented in Figures 3.6 and 3.7.

caine shipments compared with the huge, bulky shipments of coca leaves; and, although there is no hard evidence, the existence of an import duty would likely have encouraged underreporting on the part of manufacturers and importers.

Nevertheless, *Oil, Paint, and Drug Reporter* again proves useful as a starting point. It recorded cocaine imports in cases (just as it recorded coca in bales). Measured by the number of cases, cocaine imports (nearly all from Germany) increased consistently until 1895. With the emergence of a substantial American cocaine manufacturing capacity in the late 1890s, however, the quantity of imported cocaine appears to have declined.

How much cocaine was imported? Here the available records partly fail because the number of cases was very seldom accompanied by the amount of cocaine by weight in each case. Moreover, when amounts of cocaine were occasionally reported, there was great variation among them. Although most cases contained between 20 and 40 pounds of cocaine, others contained only 1 or 2 pounds, and some contained far more than 40 pounds. Estimates of "averages" from these data are inevitably problematic.

Between 1898 and 1907, however, the Commerce Department reported the dollar value of cocaine imports. Conservative estimates of cocaine imports during this period can be based on the reported dollar value. Figure 3.7 presents such estimates based on the Commerce Department data between 1898 and 1923 (the last year in which cocaine could legally be imported into the United States), which are the most reliable for that period. The data for 1887 to 1897 are based (for lack of a better alternative) on the New York import data, estimated to represent 50 percent of the true national total.

How much cocaine did Americans consume? Figure 3.8 suggests, first, that consumption totals for the early 1890s increased by at least 500 percent by the following decade. The peak of cocaine importation and manufacture in the pre-Harrison Act era was nearly 9 tons in 1903. Peak levels of more than 7 tons of cocaine were reported in 1902, 1903, 1906, and 1910. Although these estimates are conservative, they show the steady growth in the supply of cocaine.

For the companies that produced this supply, cocaine had become one of the most notable new drug products of the day, a clear sign of their industry's important place in the modern world. Along these lines, the 1893 World's Columbian Exposition featured exhibits dedicated to the technological and scientific progress of mankind, including many chemical and pharmaceutical advances. A kind of chemical hall of fame, dedicated to the most important advances in the nineteenth century (including the discovery of quinine, microorganisms and fermentation, ether, and nitroglycerin in explosives), culminated in Koller's discovery of cocaine. A decade later, at the St. Louis World's Fair, individual companies included their manufacture of cocaine as evidence of their association with modern science and medicine. Burroughs & Wellcome exhibited an enormous display of medicines and chemicals that the firm manufactured, including crystal containers full of cocaine hydrochloride. The local St. Louis–based chemical firm of Mallinckrodt Chemical Works outdid Burroughs & Wellcome with large glass globes filled with the white cocaine hydrochloride. Other indications of the importance of cocaine in drug manufacturing were less symbolic. In 1902, William Jay Schieffelin, president of the New York wholesale drug firm Schieffelin & Company, delivered an address to the American Pharmaceutical Association entitled "Advance in Pharmaceutical Manufactures During the Past Fifty Years." Among his remarks, Schieffelin noted that "fifteen years ago cocaine was sold by the grain, and now its annual consumption in America approximates 100,000 ounces. So the pharmaceutical chemist finds to-day his processes lighted by the lamp of science. The future is bright."[61]

FOUR

Selling Science
The Pharmaceutical Industry and Cocaine

The rise of cocaine use coincided with the dramatic increased capacity of the American pharmaceutical industry to produce, market, and distribute new drug products. The failure of medical control (and the end of the medical era) owed much to the power of pharmaceutical companies to promote and sell cocaine to American retailers and consumers, with or without the unqualified imprimatur of the medical profession. Bypassing physician claims to authority over the ways in which cocaine might be sold and used, manufacturers pushed the product far beyond the informal limits of medical practice. Drug makers selectively publicized medical opinion concerning cocaine, downplaying the growth of negative appraisals and expressing enthusiasm for all of its new potential applications in medical practice. Although manufacturers began with a foundation of medical research, their messages to consumers often either ignored the warnings of physicians concerning safe use or promoted uses no longer endorsed by medical consensus. Despite efforts by an emerging coalition of doctors and reformers to set standards of "appropriate" use, the pharmaceutical industry succeeded in developing a popular market for cocaine.

So-called ethical drug manufacturers occupied one end of the industry spectrum. These firms were smallest in number but included the largest manufacturers in the country. Ethical firms claimed to serve a medical market by advertising only to physicians and pharmacists; their ranks included many of the modern pharmaceutical leaders of the twentieth century, including Squibb, Eli Lilly, Upjohn, Abbott, and Parke, Davis.

The remainder of the pharmaceutical industry in the 1890s included an enormous number of firms selling patent medicines. These medicines were not actually patented, but they were protected by trademark (and are consequently referred to by some as *proprietary remedies*).[1] Like their ethical counterparts, patent medicine makers advertised and sold their products through drug wholesalers and to pharmacists. Patent medicine makers, however, also advertised and sold products directly to the public. The *Pharmaceutical Era Druggists Directory* listed 5,398 drug manufacturers at the turn of the century; most were in the patent medicine business.[2]

When cocaine was introduced in the 1880s, the similarities between ethical and patent medicine enterprises outweighed the differences. Because cocaine could be purchased without a prescription, influencing the attitudes of retail druggists was important for establishing confidence in the product. Patent medicine and ethical drug firms had to convince druggists not only that they should keep cocaine and cocaine products in stock but that they also should recommend them to their customers. Ethical houses could avoid the scrutiny of physicians while maintaining the posture of not dealing directly with the consumer. Patent medicine manufacturers acknowledged more openly that they bypassed physician authority, making many additional appeals directly to the American consumer.

Two characteristics of the late-nineteenth-century drug market facilitated aggressive promotion. First, companies introducing new drugs faced few or no legal controls over their claims concerning uses, benefits, and effects. Laws concerning the purity of drugs existed in only a few states, and political pressures limited their enforcement. The first effective nationwide regulatory efforts appeared only with the Pure Food and Drug Act of 1906 and the creation of the American Medical Association Council on Pharmacy and Chemistry.[3]

Second, no single acknowledged authority could define for consumers what was and was not a legitimate use for cocaine. Among physicians, traditional medical practice was being challenged by practitioners of alternative medicine such as homeopathy and eclecticism as well as by a host of fringe practitioners and quacks.[4] Many consumers avoided medical advice altogether and opted for the purchase of their own medicines.

Parke, Davis & Company: Selling the Power of Cocaine

Among the ethical firms in the United States, none had a larger stake in the success of cocaine than Parke, Davis. In securing a market for its product, the company discarded an older, conservative version of the pharmaceutical manufacturer function and adopted innovative business practices. These practices would not only popularize cocaine, they would form the foundation of the twentieth-century drug business.

Before the 1880s, ethical pharmaceutical manufacturers traditionally viewed their enterprise as a reactive one, responding to the demand for certain products by druggists and doctors. Much of the product offered by older houses consisted of raw materials because both doctors and druggists still compounded their own remedies.[5]

The firm of Parke, Davis began as a pharmaceutical manufacturer in this traditional mold. Established in 1866 in Detroit by Hervey Parke and Dr. Samuel Duffield, the firm of Duffield, Parke & Company remained small and unimportant during its first years of operation. Although it served Detroit and the surrounding region, it presented no competition to manufacturers in New York and Philadelphia, the centers of the pharmaceutical industry. A few years later, a young salesman named George S. Davis used money he borrowed from his mother to buy part of the existing firm. After Dr. Duffield (for unrelated reasons) left the company, it became known as Parke, Davis.[6]

Neither Parke nor Davis had any medical or pharmaceutical experience, an unusual circumstance in an age when many large ethical firms were headed by individuals with experience in one or both fields.[7] In every other respect, the owners, Parke and Davis, were quite different. Hervey Parke, the older of the two men, was a quiet and conservative man who believed in running a traditional drug manufactory. It was George S. Davis who revolutionized the way in which the company did business. Although younger and less experienced in the business than Parke, he possessed a vision of the capacity of pharmaceutical firms to create demand for new products. As an employee of the firm recalled, Davis was "the promotion man" and largely responsible for the company's dramatic growth. In the memory of company employees, Davis had an "aggressiveness" that "was irresistible," with methods of salesmanship which turned Parke, Davis into a pharmaceutical powerhouse.[8]

Davis' conception of the pharmaceutical business was that of a salesman. To Davis, the object of the drug business was the same as every other type of manufacturing enterprise: to sell its products. Although Davis understood the irony that "Parke, Davis & Company is an organization of business men engaged in teaching the medical profession therapeutics," he embraced this role.[9] For Davis, the most attractive products for the company were those the firm could help to popularize, thus creating and controlling new markets. The company officially called such products "new remedies" and advertised them as such. One of the first new remedies was coca.

In selling cocaine to the medical profession, the first task of ethical firms such as Parke, Davis was to ensure that positive medical research was communicated to as many pharmacists and physicians as possible. To that end, Parke, Davis established a publishing enterprise in the 1870s, headed by George Davis, to disseminate information about the drug products of the firm. Cocaine was one of the first major drug discoveries to benefit from the ability of drug makers to communicate directly with prescribers. Parke, Davis publications such as the *Medical Age, New Preparations, Bulletin of Pharmacy,* and the *Therapeutic Gazette* reprinted articles from New York and Philadelphia medical journals.[10] *Medical Age,* "A Semi-Monthly Journal of Medicine and Surgery," published more than twenty research reports on cocaine in 1885. Published research from the *Edinburgh Medical Journal, Medical Times, Philadelphia Medical News, New York Medical News, Journal of Inebriety, Journal of the American Medical Association, Medical Record,* and many others found its way into the pages of Parke, Davis journals.[11]

Through the efforts of pharmaceutical firms, articles that might otherwise have had a limited distribution received much wider attention. One report might eventually appear in several publications, such as the work of Louisville physician E. R. Palmer. Palmer had originally reported the successful treatment of alcoholism with coca in the late 1870s in the *Louisville Medical News.* Parke, Davis thought the article positive enough to reprint in the *Therapeutic Gazette.* Likewise, when the William R. Warner Company of Philadelphia published a monograph entitled *Coca* in 1885, they also described Palmer's work to the thousands of eastern physicians who would probably not otherwise have learned about Palmer's research.[12]

The pinnacle of the reprint effort was reached with the publication by Parke, Davis of *The Pharmacology of the Newer Materia Medica* (1892). Ostensibly a reference publication, the book featured summaries of journal articles describing the many Parke, Davis products. Essentially an annotated bibliography of work on Parke, Davis specialties, the book featured a staggering 240 pages on coca and cocaine. Although by 1892 many medical studies had described cases of cocaine abuse and warned of the potential dangers of the drug, Parke, Davis showed a clear editorial bias against negative results; articles on the dangers of cocaine comprised only 3 of the 240 pages.[13]

Manufacturers not only downplayed negative reporting on cocaine, in some instances they continued to reprint old medical studies long after the studies had ceased to represent mainstream medical opinion. The New York wholesale and manufacturing firm of McKesson & Robbins included in its 1885 drug catalog a reference (uncredited) to the work of William Hammond: "a prominent physician considers cocaine a means of curing the opium habit if properly used. He has never seen a habit formed by its use, and classes the drug rather with tea and coffee than with opium in this respect." Hammond's assertions about the use of cocaine in treating addiction, and its safety, were never wholly supported by physicians. Remarkably, McKesson & Robbins continued to use Hammond's conclusions in its catalogs through 1894. At that time Hammond's views were widely discredited, Hammond himself was retired from active practice, and he had said nothing about cocaine for eight years.[14]

As Parke, Davis introduced its group of new remedies in the 1870s, a number of physicians initially accused the company of practicing quackery by promoting new drug products themselves rather than waiting for favorable medical studies. In many instances the origin and physiological actions of these new products were not revealed in order to protect the company's investment. Critics pointed out that for an ethical firm to advertise new products in this manner was too much like the marketing practices of patent medicine manufacturers. Edward R. Squibb claimed that "advertising is at its best misleading. At its worst it is the worst form of quackery — made up of garbled quotations, fraudulent claims and lying statements mixed with a little truth. It is astonishing how much fraud, error, humbug, and lies a little truth can carry."[15] A report in the *New England Medical Monthly* accused Parke, Davis of "trying to overrun our materia medica." Its author concluded, "I express, as a member of society, and as a practitioner, the belief that I cherish, that their [Parke, Davis] arguments are unsound, their methods improper, and the extensive advertising is reprehensible, as is the very reprehensible practice of the patent medicine quackery."[16] These admonitions led George Davis, by the early 1880s, to the conclusion that promotion had to be backed by the appearance of scientific rigor.

In March 1881, Parke, Davis formally established a pharmacological laboratory. Its goal, according to the company, was "to do botanical, historical, and pharmacologic work on the materia medica and to submit it in the form of literature to the *Therapeutic Gazette* for publication for the use of the medical profession."[17] To that end, Parke, Davis became the first pharmaceutical firm to employ a scientific staff. Among the first hired were chemist Albert B. Lyons, botanist Henry Hurd Rusby, and physician Francis Edward Stewart.[18] Many of their contributions were genuine scientific advances. Lyons, for example, helped Parke, Davis become the first company to standardize the strength of its pharmaceutical preparations.[19] Stewart was hired by the firm to write medical reports, called *working bulletins,* on the firm's products. With Stewart providing credibility, the firm hoped its future advertising might be viewed as evidence of scientific progress rather than quackery. Stewart himself suggested that "before the introduction of the working bulletin system the publication of this information in medical journal advertisement was called the 'worst form of quackery.' When published in the form of 'working bulletins' it was credited as valuable research work and the demand for the new remedies grew rapidly to the advantage of all concerned."[20]

Every member of the Parke, Davis scientific staff worked to increase the visibility of coca and cocaine. Rusby's studies on the origin and characteristics of coca were reprinted widely, earning him a reputation as one of the leading experts on coca.[21] Head chemist Lyons was a frequent contributor of articles on cocaine to the pages of the *American Journal of Pharmacy*.[22] Early in 1885, Lyons published in the *Therapeutic Gazette* the results of a comparative study of cocaine which was on the market. Not surprisingly, he rated Parke, Davis cocaine the best available followed in order by E. Merck & Company, W. H. Schieffelin & Company, a German product distributed by Lehn & Fink, Squibb, and McKesson & Robbins. The worst of the products was distributed by the firm of Glover & Nichol and consisted of pure sodium carbonate with not a trace of cocaine.[23]

An early effort to stimulate public interest was a Stewart-authored medical monograph on the fluid extract of coca. In addition to describing its potential benefits, the monograph concluded that "complaint has been made, and not without foundation, that a large proportion of the coca leaves offered for sale in the United States is worthless."[24] Stewart claimed that Parke, Davis had solved this "problem" by obtaining its coca directly from Bolivia and manufacturing a preparation of standardized strength.

Both Rusby and Stewart had contracts that allowed for a commission on the sales of products they helped introduce. When Parke, Davis developed coca leaf cigars and cigarettes, Stewart reminded the firm that he considered himself responsible for the idea. Davis wrote back to Stewart allowing that a commission would be paid "providing that you will undertake to write up in such a way that will provide us proper material in the way of medical articles for circulation."[25] Stewart rewarded the Parke, Davis investment with the publication of "Coca Leaf Cigars and Cigarettes" in the *Philadelphia Medical Times*.

The firm also distributed cocaine free or at low cost to physicians in exchange for contributed reports on the drug's effectiveness. In his correspondence with the firm, Stewart was asked to supply individual Philadelphia physicians with cocaine.[26] Stewart also offered at the conclusion of his *Philadelphia Medical Times* to send samples of coca leaf cigars, free of charge, to any physician who would "test them, and publish the results."[27] C. N. Anderson, hired by Davis in the early 1880s, was certain that company promotional efforts worked to encourage research and influence physicians. While attending the St. Louis World's Fair and pitching a new disinfectant, Anderson met the head doctor of the fair. A great fan of Parke, Davis, the doctor told Anderson that he had experimented with the therapeutic use of cocaine early in his career. Sending $1.25 for a pound of coca leaves, the young doctor soon received his money back, along with 5 pounds of leaves and an encouraging letter from George Davis. "This," the doctor declared, "was the action of a BIG house."[28]

Despite the Parke, Davis efforts, negative reports on cocaine appeared in medical and pharmaceutical journals. Reports of cocaine poisoning were particularly troubling because the safety of cocaine was critical to its medical appeal. Fortunately, medical theorizing provided the manufacturers with a credible explanation: that these reactions resulted from impurities and by-products in the cocaine. Cocaine manufacturers seconded this point of view and assured customers that *their* cocaine remained free of these potentially hazardous ingredients. In its own trade journal, Parke, Davis noted that "our cocaine hydrochlorate must be free from excess of acid and from foreign and dangerous alkaloids whose presence accounts for the cocaine-intoxications and fatalities reported."[29] With each vial of its cocaine, C. F. Boehringer & Soehne furnished a "test of purity" to its customers, a test that was undoubtedly rarely performed but implied safety.[30]

Parke, Davis established the potential power of the modern pharmaceutical industry, and cocaine was among the first drugs to benefit. The newly proactive marketing strategies promoted rapid diffusion of information, diluted the effects of negative stories, and established loyalty among those who distributed cocaine directly to the public (especially retail druggists).

Patent Medicines and the Popularization of Cocaine

Patent medicine manufacturers formed the largest segment of the pharmaceutical industry, far outnumbering ethical firms and holding the largest share of the drug market. The Bureau of the Census *Manufactures 1914* recorded that the value of all "druggists' preparations" totaled forty-eight million dollars, just under half the value of "patent medicines and compounds."[31] The importance of the patent medicine industry went beyond sales; its hold on consumer loyalty represented a formidable challenge to physicians and ethical firms alike. Many consumers, unwilling or unable to seek the help of a physician, placed their trust in the makers of products on drugstore shelves. The visibility of patent medicines, which secured them an important place in drug manufacturing, was itself secured by some of the most active and innovative advertising of the era (Figure 4.1).

Patent medicines undeniably helped to shape consumer attitudes toward cocaine by making the drug's uses and characteristics more familiar. They created and sustained a market for cocaine only marginally dependent on medical direction or control. Even the briefest of historical reviews of the history of cocaine ac-

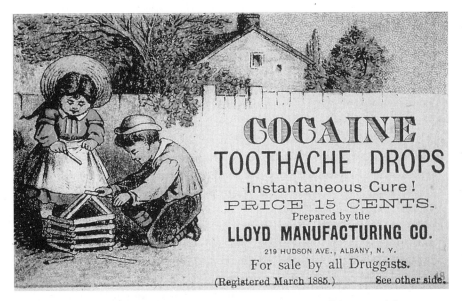

Figure 4.1. Patent medicine advertisement. The earliest patent medicines containing cocaine utilized the drug's anesthetic powers. Cocaine Toothache Drops, according to this advertisement, were registered in March 1885, just five months after Koller's dramatic announcement. National Library of Medicine.

knowledge the importance of the patent medicine trade, yet two major points of contention still require critical examination.

First, many historical accounts express skepticism that any therapeutic claim advertised by patent medicine manufacturers was made in good faith. These claims are construed as deliberately false representations by manufacturers who understood that their products would, in fact, do no good at all.[32] The medical wisdom of the late twentieth century has tended to reinforce this view by demonstrating that such products could not "cure" the diseases for which they were intended. Other historical studies, however, find outright fraud to have been the exception rather than the rule. Instead, many patent medicine manufacturers seem to have borrowed heavily from traditional medical practice (while suggesting to their customers the irrelevance of a physician's counsel).[33] The cocaine experience lies somewhere in between these two opposing perspectives. Outrageous and dangerous claims exposed some consumers to considerable risk, whereas many other products were merely extensions of mainstream medical thought.

A second, much-debated aspect of the patent medicine business concerns the role of the consumer. Many studies assume that manufacturers secretly added drugs such as cocaine to their preparations without informing the public. The consumer-as-dupe model originated in Progressive Era crusades against patent medicines. Progressive reformers portrayed the pharmaceutical industry as they did many other large corporate interests: poisoners of the health and welfare of the American population and conscience-less pursuers of profit. Cocaine has always fit this model quite nicely; later historians (influenced by more contemporary attitudes toward cocaine) would suggest that any use of a drug as dangerous as cocaine must have been hidden from an unwitting public. Actual practices show that many manufacturers made no effort to hide the cocaine in their product but rather stressed its presence. The development and sale of the two best-known coca/cocaine products, Coca-Cola and Vin Mariani, illustrate this part of the patent medicine enterprise.

The Medical Roots of Popular Products:
Coca-Cola and Vin Mariani

Every history of cocaine has something to say about Coca-Cola because Coca-Cola developed into one of the most popular products in the world with a well-documented early history. Yet most historical accounts have misinterpreted the relationship between cocaine and Coca-Cola. Some accounts suggest that the drink was only a thinly disguised means for cocaine seekers to obtain the drug. Because "even Coca-Cola had it," cocaine use must have been widespread and unrestrained. Other accounts have gone in the opposite direction, asserting either that the drink never contained cocaine or that its presence was accidental.

Ample historical evidence illustrates the shortcomings of both viewpoints. Coca-Cola not only contained cocaine, its raison d'être was to serve as an appetizing vehicle for both the stimulant and therapeutic properties of coca. John Pemberton, the creator of Coca-Cola, was an Atlanta pharmacist who also did some manufacturing for a limited market. Among Pemberton's products was a coca wine, which he called Peruvian Wine Coca. The city of Atlanta adopted prohibition in 1886, forcing Pemberton to seek an alternative to Peruvian Wine Coca which would contain no alcohol. The syrup that resulted from his experiments he called Coca-Cola.[34] From the beginning, Pemberton intended this product to serve a medical market albeit through a delicious fountain drink.

In its early advertising, Coca-Cola not only openly acknowledged its coca content, it ardently invoked accepted medical knowledge of coca to make its sales pitch. In 1896, the *National Druggist*, a St. Louis publication, ran its first advertisement for Coca-Cola:

It seems to be a law of nature that the more valuable and efficacious a drug is, the nastier and more unpleasant its taste. It is therefore quite a triumph over nature that the Coca-Cola Co. of Atlanta, Ga., have achieved in their success in robbing both coca leaves and the kola nut of the exceedingly nauseous and disagreeable taste while retaining their wonderful medicinal properties, and the power of restoring vitality and raising the spirits of the weary and debilitated. Not only have they done this, but by some subtle alchemy they have made them the basis of one of the most delightful, cheering, and invigorating of fountain drinks.[35]

Coca-Cola continued this type of advertising appeal into the first decade of the twentieth century (Figure 4.2). A 1907 advertisement in the same journal made fewer therapeutic claims, but it did discuss the company's use of the coca leaf:

They know, too, that the slightly exhilarating effects are no more harmful than a cup of tea or coffee, but make Coca-Cola the ideal, as well as the most popular, of all beverages, in these days of strenuous methods in both work and play. To secure the properties used in genuine Coca-Cola, nature's choicest gift to two hemispheres must be found and transported across both mountains and seas. High in the Andes, the Peruvians endure severest privations by chewing the coca leaf.[36]

The company traded upon the therapeutic potency of coca, but its product contained only small amounts of cocaine. Although the formula of Coca-Cola remained a closely guarded secret, most published accounts presumed that Pemberton employed coca in his product, a presumption confirmed in 1993 with the publication of the original formula by Mark Pendergrast. The formula discovered by Pendergrast called for the addition of 4 ounces of "F. E. Coco," which, despite the misspelling, referred to the fluid extract of coca.[37]

Pemberton was enthusiastic but did not bring Coca-Cola financial success. As Richard S. Tedlow commented, "if the drink had remained in the hands of John Styth Pemberton, it would have gone the way of his Extract of Styllinger and Globe Flower Cough Syrup."[38] Instead, the company came under the control of Asa G. Candler in 1891. Candler made no changes in the formula of Coca-Cola or its therapeutic claims. Candler did push sales of Coca-Cola, which went from $12,400 in 1890 to $519,200 in 1900. Even more remarkably, sales rose to $5,505,900 in the next decade, indicating a truly national market for the soft drink.[39]

The phenomenal success of Coca-Cola gave rise to a host of imitators, particularly in the South, where Coca-Cola had its first success. Of the ten soft drinks containing cocaine mentioned in the American Medical Association *Nostrums and Quackery,* three were manufactured in Atlanta; two in Birmingham, Alabama; one each in Athens, Georgia; New Orleans; Cincinnati; Canton, Ohio;

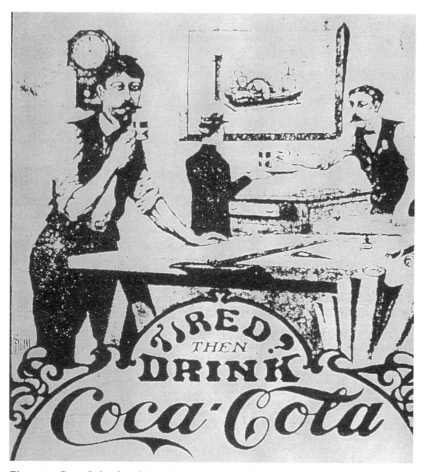

Figure 4.2. Coca-Cola advertisement. Surviving pre-1920 advertisements for Coca-Cola emphasized the connection between the drink and its therapeutic effect. Here "tired" and "exhausted" draftsmen take a drink and presumably notice the immediate benefits of coca-cocaine.

and Chicago.[40] Scores of Coca-Cola imitators, with names like Cafe-Coca, Kos-Kola, Kola-Ade, Celery-Cola, Koca-Nola, Wiseola, Rococola, Vani-Kola, and Koke, competed for a part of the lucrative soft drink market. The composition of most Coca-Cola competitors followed a similar pattern as well. Most used fluid extract of coca in largely the same proportions as Coca-Cola. Consequently, most contained extremely small amounts of cocaine (see Table 4.1).

The promotion of Coca-Cola remained consistent even as sales soared. The therapeutic underpinnings of Coca-Cola as a tonic and stimulant were, as noted,

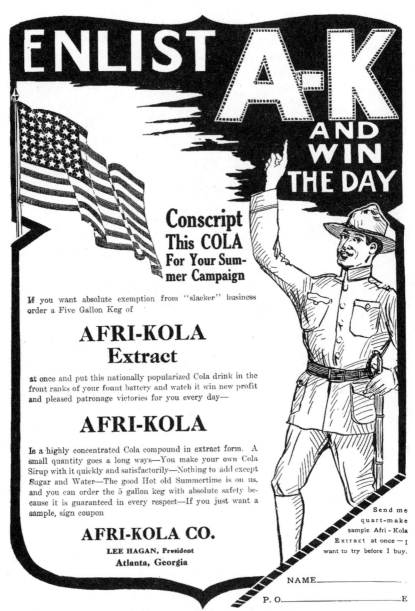

Figure 4.3. Afri-Kola advertisement. Before 1920, a staggering number of coca soft drinks came and went, in fierce competition for soda fountain space. In a competitive environment, Afri-Kola looked to secure its own niche in the trade. By the time this advertisement appeared in 1917, Afri-Kola had joined most other soft drinks in becoming "de-cocainized." Courtesy of the American Institute of the History of Pharmacy.

left essentially unchanged by Candler in the years after he purchased the company in 1891. Over time, the connection between the therapeutic use of Coca-Cola as a tonic and advertising that emphasized the product as delicious and refreshing blurred a bit. Competitors of Coca-Cola largely chose to emphasize general tonic properties rather than specific therapeutic claims (Figure 4.3). The Wiseola slogan referred to the drink as "sparkling, refreshing, delicious, invigorating"; Kos-Kola was "refreshing — healthful — invigorating — delicious"; Celery-Cola claimed to be "exhilarating, refreshing, pure and sold round the world"; and Koca-Nola billed itself as "the Great Tonic Drink."[41]

Before Coca-Cola, coca wines occupied the most prominent position among coca/cocaine products. Mortimer's physician survey revealed that among 276 physicians who employed coca in their practice, only 15 used a solid extract of coca, 20 used coca leaves, 104 used the fluid extract, and 229 used coca wine. Coca wine, employed by 83 percent of Mortimer's physicians, was clearly the coca preparation of choice for physicians.[42] It was also the preparation of choice for the public; cocaine appeared more often in coca wines than any other form during the 1880s and 1890s.

Vin Mariani was the first and most popular of the coca wines. Mariani & Company typified the close relationship between some patent medicine manufacturers and physicians. Mariani claimed to advertise only to physicians, echoing the practices of ethical firms. Mariani devised numerous promotions for its product lines, including the publication of its own periodical, *Mariani's Coca Leaf: An Occasional Review for Physicians Advocating The Rational Uses of Coca,* "mailed free to physicians upon request"[43] (Figure 4.4). Mariani also used an early type of celebrity endorsement, clearly designed to appeal to an educated, professional constituency rather than a mass market. The aggressive pursuit of medical favor resulted in the company being able to boast of having the written endorsement of more than seven thousand physicians.

Like Coca-Cola, Vin Mariani inspired a host of imitators. The peak of coca wine popularity came in the early 1890s, when the catalog of New York wholesale dealer Charles N. Crittenton listed nineteen different brands of coca wine available to the public.[44] The *Druggists' Circular Price List* for 1900 listed the following coca wines: Bartlett & Plummer's, Burgundia, Cushing's, Frazer's, Funk's, Health Restorative, Kleinschmidt's, Lambert's, Liebig's, Llewellyn's, Mariani's, McKelway's, Metcalf's, Milhau's, Morgan's, Neergaard's, Riker's, Robinson's, Schieffelin's, and Von Hauff's. Although it is impossible to determine the precise composition of each product, they were probably quite variable. Some manufacturers of coca wines simply dosed their product with cocaine rather than a fluid extract of coca, coming up with a cheaper and more potent

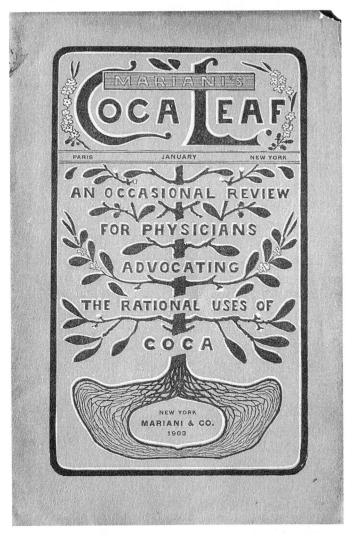

Figure 4.4. Mariani's Coca Leaf. Some patent medicines took pride in their popularity among physicians, despite doing much of their business directly with the public. Few nurtured that relationship as assiduously as Mariani and Company. For a short time, the company published an American journal for doctors interested in "the rational uses of coca." Courtesy of the Lloyd Library and Museum, Cincinnati.

product in one step. In its advertisements, the Mariani Company acknowledged the competition and implored its customers to avoid products made with "cheap wine and cocaine"[45] (Figure 4.5).

Coca, Cocaine, and the Variety of Patent Medicines

Tonic preparations, soft drinks, and coca wines dominated the lists of coca and cocaine products. Long before coca and cocaine appeared in the 1880s, dozens of "restoratives" and "invigorators" filled drugstore cases and shelves. In many instances, manufacturers simply added coca to an already successful and established line of tonics. The Liebig Company, for example, already had a successful, nationally distributed product line of beef compounds, such as Iron and Beef. As endorsements of the therapeutic value of coca appeared in medical and pharmaceutical journals, the Liebig Company simply added some fluid extract of coca and developed another product for its line, which they called Coca Beef Compound.[46] The Lambert Company expanded its line of medicinal wines with prod-

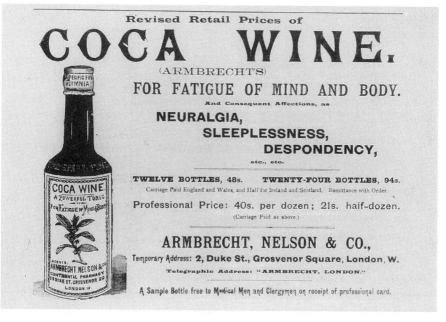

Figure 4.5. This advertisement for Lambrecht's Coca Wine originally appeared in the April 1889 issue of *The Illustrated Medical News* (London). Of the therapeutic claims, only that for sleeplessness was unusual. Note that the manufacturer concludes by offering free sample bottles to medical men and clergymen. National Library of Medicine.

ucts such as Lambert's Wine of Coca with Peptonate Iron and Extract of Cod Liver Oil.

Most patent medicine advertising emphasized the tonic and stimulant properties of cocaine. A St. Louis firm that manufactured a product called Cocarettes, made with tobacco and coca leaves, listed "Ten Reasons Why Cocarettes Should Be Used By All Smokers" (Figure 4.6). Included on the list were: "Coca is the finest nerve tonic and exhilarator ever discovered"; "Coca stimulates the brain to great activity and gives tone and vigor to the entire system."[47]

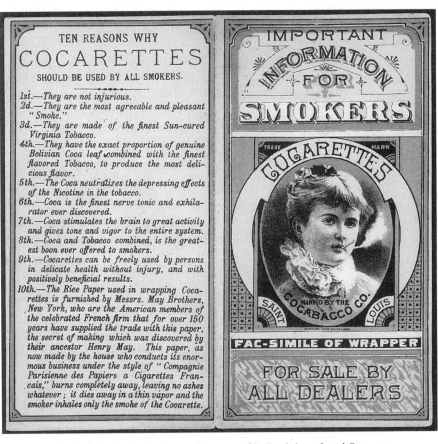

Figure 4.6. Around 1885, the Cocabacco Company of St. Louis introduced Cocarettes, combining coca and tobacco in one of the few commercial uses of coca for smoking purposes. This advertisement explains the therapeutic benefits in great detail, while assuring consumers a pleasurable smoke. The addition of coca to already popular products was common practice among manufacturers. Courtesy of the Strong Museum, Rochester, N.Y.

Even in products in which cocaine was a relatively small part of a formula, its tonic properties were highlighted in advertising. Nyal's Compound Extract of Damiana, sold as an aphrodisiac, noted that coca "is a muscle tonic, and exalts the intellectual facilities." The label of Coca Calisaya claimed that it could sustain "the strength under extreme physical exertion."[48] Many such cures appear to have traded upon the popular reputation of cocaine without actually using a significant amount of the drug in the product.

As the rather unappealing appellation given to Lambert's Wine of Coca with Peptonate Iron and Extract of Cod Liver Oil suggests, many patent preparations were intended for a medical market. Although Lambert employed coca, other manufacturers used small amounts of cocaine. The G. F. Harvey Company of Saratoga Springs, New York, manufactured several medical products using cocaine as an ingredient. One, a "stomachic sedative" tablet, contained about 5 milligrams of cocaine. Similarly, the William A. Webster antivomiting tablets contained 4 milligrams of cocaine. Cocaine became, in fact, a small but popular ingredient in many brands of voice and throat tablets. The Harvey Company also manufactured two types of voice tablets (one chocolate coated) which each contained less than 1 milligram of cocaine.[49]

The other significant therapeutic category among the first patent medicine preparations were various "habit cures." These cures were inspired by the medical use of cocaine in treating alcoholism and opiate addiction. The most common of these appear to have been tobacco habit cures, such as Elders' Celebrated Tobacco Specific, Tobacco Bullets, and Wonder Workers. As with the ethical manufacturers of drugs and medicines, the most interesting feature of the claims made for these cures by the patent medicine industry was less what they said than the length of time the industry was willing to say it. Patent medicine manufacturers embraced the positive recommendations of doctors in the 1880s and early 1890s but then ignored the emerging negative view in the mid 1890s and early 1900s.

Charles L. Mitchell of Philadelphia, himself a physician, created a product called Coca-Bola, a chewing paste with cocaine. On the front of the package Mitchell cited an 1886 study by fellow Philadelphia physician William Waugh. Waugh's study suggested, as did many others in 1886, that cocaine could be useful in the treatment of the tobacco, alcohol, and opium habits.[50] Mitchell, however, continued to use Waugh's study for at least two decades after it was published — and well after medical studies had denounced the use of cocaine in the treatment of addictions.

Although the first generation of patent medicines containing coca or cocaine was remarkably varied, some general features stand out. These early preparations were, in many instances, not enough to create or satisfy habitual users who consumed 500 to 1,000 milligrams of cocaine in a single day (even more in some cases). On the other hand, many were potent enough to have a noticeable effect on users (a contemporary "line" of cocaine might average about 50 milligrams).

The soft drinks on the list, in particular, appear to have contained very little cocaine. Any habit-forming potential probably derived from their caffeine, not cocaine content (Table 4.1).

Just as physicians often used coca instead of cocaine, the first generation of patent medicines contained coca as often as cocaine. The wholesale catalogs of the Chicago firm of Peter Van Schaack & Sons (one of the largest in the Midwest) reflect the early importance of coca products. Its 1888 catalog included nineteen products that could positively be identified as containing either coca or cocaine. Most were coca wines or tonic compounds with coca. In only three cases did the manufacturing process involve the addition of cocaine rather than coca or a coca extract.[51]

TABLE 4.1
Cocaine Content of Patent Medicines

Product	Cocaine Content[a]
Wiseola	>1
Celery-Cola	>1
Koca-Nola	>1
Dick's Toothache Gum	3
Allenbury's Throat Pastilles	3
Liquid Peptonoids with Coca	3
Kola Coca	5
Vin Mariani	6–8
Kola Cardinette[b]	9
Maltine with Coca	9
Esencia de Coca (Parke, Davis)	25
Coca Cordial (Parke, Davis)	30
Metcalf Coca Wine	32
Coke Extract[c]	39
Nichol's Compound Coca Cordial	62
Coca-Bola	710

SOURCES: John Phillips Street, *The Composition of Certain Patent and Proprietary Medicines* (Chicago: American Medical Association, 1917). For Celery-Cola, Koca-Nola, and Coke Extract, see *Nostrums and Quackery* (American Medical Association, 1912). For Esencia de Coca and Coca Cordial, see Parke, Davis & Company Collection. For Kola Cardinette, see Bureau of Chemistry hearing 89 (February 25, 1908).
  [a]Data are in milligrams per ounce.
  [b]Kola Cardinette reported only the coca content on their package label.
  [c]Coke Extract was likely designed as a syrup to be mixed with carbonated water, resulting in a soft drink with a potency comparable to that of the others listed here.

The first generation of coca/cocaine products was also the largest. The absolute number peaked quickly and declined gradually. The wholesale catalogs of the Van Schaack Company reflect this pattern. The nineteen products in its 1888 catalog were the most Van Schaack ever stocked. The decline in the availability of these early products was gradual but unmistakable; only twelve of the nineteen products were carried in the Van Schaack 1900 catalog, then nine in 1904 and seven in 1907.[52]

At first glance, it is surprising that the absolute number of coca/cocaine products from the patent medicine industry declined as the overall amount of cocaine consumed through all sources (including patent medicines) increased. The seemingly conflicting trends may be explained by noting the rise of a final group of patent medicines in the mid 1890s: the asthma and catarrh cures.

The Catarrh Cures

The appearance in the 1890s Van Schaack wholesale catalogs of Agnew's and Birney's catarrh cures, two of the most popular national brands containing cocaine, may be taken as a small but important indicator of a new phase in the packaging of cocaine. As the medical market decreased in importance, some manufacturers found success in selling cheap and easy-to-use cocaine products such as the catarrh cures. In most instances, the cocaine was taken by sniffing, a practice that rapidly became the most prominent means of administration.

The catarrh cure began as an extension of medical practice, reflecting the popularity of cocaine inhalation as a means of dealing with sinus irritation. In 1888, Dr. Nathan S. Tucker introduced Tucker's Asthma Specific, a stronger cocaine solution than Az-Ma-Syde. Tucker's Asthma Specific sold at a relatively high cost of $12.50 for an atomizer, descriptive pamphlet, and 4 ounces of the solution (which contained slightly more than 1,800 milligrams of cocaine). Despite a retail price far higher than a comparable quantity of pure cocaine hydrochloride, the Asthma Specific sold quite well. An investigation revealed that Tucker purchased between 256 and 384 ounces of cocaine a month from one manufacturer.[53] Over twelve months, this amount of cocaine would have allowed Tucker to manufacture and distribute between 50,000 and 80,000 units of his Specific, worth $625,000 to $1,000,000. Tucker himself boasted of his Specific: "we supply the whole world with it."[54]

Gradually, less expensive cocaine snuffs supplanted the cocaine sprays. The first of the popular cocaine snuffs appeared in drugstores in the early 1890s. In 1895, the *National Druggist* offered its readers a cure for a "Bad Cold" which involved the use of an atomizer with a 1 percent solution of cocaine. The journal also included an alternative remedy of a snuff containing almost 5 percent cocaine.

Most of the cocaine snuffs/catarrh cures followed the same basic formula.[55] Parke, Davis offered readers of its drug journals a typical formula for 1 ounce of catarrh snuff, with 4 percent cocaine:

Sodium Bicarbonate	10 grains
Magnesium carbonate	15 grains
Menthol	5 grains
Cocaine muriate	20 grains
Sugar of milk	450 grains

The composition of most catarrh snuffs followed the same rules as the Parke, Davis formula, the key variable being the amount of cocaine involved.[56] The formula book of a Michigan retail druggist described a less potent snuff while still adhering to the basic formula:

Sodium bismuth	2 grains
Magnesium carbonate	3 grains
Cocaine	4 grains
Sugar of milk	720 grains

The composition of these catarrh snuffs represented an extension of, rather than a challenge to, mainstream medical wisdom. The manufacture of catarrh snuffs merely offered cheap relief to a wider audience. Moreover, the cocaine content of the cures, although higher than most products on the market, rarely exceeded 5 percent. A product such as Ryno's Hay Fever and Catarrh Remedy, which the Bureau of Chemistry found to contain 99.95 percent cocaine, stood alone.[57]

The composition of catarrh snuffs also fit very nicely with the requirements of manufacturers who sought to sell their product to the widest possible market. First, the manufacture of such preparations involved minimal cost because they consisted primarily of inexpensive sugar of milk (lactose). The lactose allowed manufacturers to keep the cost of the product to the consumer fairly low and still make a huge profit. Most of the leading brands sold at retail for 50¢, although some brands offered a range of product sizes as cheap as 25¢ and as expensive as $1. Second, catarrh snuffs were convenient and effective products for consumers. Their overall cocaine content, relative to other medicines with coca or cocaine, was certainly much higher (Table 4.2). Such figures represent estimates; the variable numbers reflect changing composition.[58]

By 1900, catarrh cures had emerged as the most notorious cocaine product, closely associated with the popular, nonmedical consumption of the drug. Manufacturers of the leading brands, in contrast to many of the coca tonic makers,

TABLE 4.2
*Cocaine in the Leading Catarrh and
Asthma Remedies*

Product	Amount of Cocaine [a]
Agnew's Catarrhal Powder	500
Anglo-American Catarrhal	270
Birney's Catarrh Powder	585–1250
Cole's Catarrh Cure	850–1175
Crown Catarrh Powder	570–850
Gray's Catarrh Powder	470
Instant Catarrh Relief	710
Az-Ma-Syde	290
Tucker's Asthma Specific	230–450

SOURCES: John Phillips Street, *The Composition of Certain Patent and Proprietary Medicines* (Chicago: American Medical Association, 1917).
[a]Data are in milligrams of cocaine per ounce of product.

typically specialized in that one product. In Chicago, Birney's Catarrhal Powder Company, for example, made Birney's Catarrh Cure, one of the nation's most popular brands. Others, such as the Anglo-American Medicine Company in New York (makers of Agnew's Catarrh Cure), produced a limited number of additional products. The Standard Remedy Company of Boston produced several different cocaine-based catarrh cures, including A No. 1 Catarrh Cure, Opal Catarrh Powder, Ruby Catarrh Powder, and Standard Catarrh Powder. Different regions of the country had different leading brands; in Chicago, the two leading cures were Birney's and Crown Catarrh Powder. The Christian Civic League of Maine suggested that in Portland, they found cocaine "vended in the form of cold cures, etc. The form, exceeding all others combined, is I.C.R. or 'Instant Catarrh Relief.' This contains 2½% of hydrochlorate cocaine and is manufactured at New Durham, NH."[59]

The hyperbole and energy of catarrh cure advertising also contrast with the more restrained opinions expressed by most physicians concerning cocaine. Az-Ma-Syde noted on its label that "a prominent practicing physician has discovered and successfully used for the past few years this wonderful remedy known as AZ-MA-SYDE." The makers of Az-Ma-Syde were not shy about the curative power of their product over asthma: "On a Guarantee We Will Cure ASTHMA or Ask No Pay. We have a cure for asthma that is POSITIVE. We know this to be a fact. It is not an irritating powder or pastille to be burned, or any of the thousand-and-one remedies that have been the source of such keen disappointment."[60] Even more questionable was the claim by the Cole Medicine Co. that its catarrh snuff was perfectly safe. In a circular to druggists, the company announced that "consumers do not become 'dopes' or 'wrecks'; on the contrary, thousands of instances are known where the cure had done perfect work along the lines intended."[61]

Manufacturers encouraged repeated, long-term use of their products. The makers of Az-Ma-Syde recommended that "to cure Asthma use . . . Az-Ma-Syde Atomizer, three times a day, and during each attack."[62] A circular for Ryno's Hay Fever and Catarrh Remedy (which contained nothing but cocaine) advised that for its use in "hay fever, rose cold, influenza, or whenever the nose is 'stuffed-up,' red and sore," the remedy should be employed "two to ten times a day, or oftener if really necessary." For "chronic catarrh" Ryno noted that the remedy should be employed two or three times a day, but that "this disease is often very intractable, sometimes requiring several months to cure."[63]

Catarrh cures seldom revealed their cocaine content. Advertising for Ryno's Remedy failed to mention that the product contained any cocaine even though it contained nothing but the drug![64] Birney's Catarrh Cure, perhaps the most well known of these, also revealed nothing about its cocaine content. Although many users understood fully the composition of these cures, some embarked on a lengthy program of treatment and then struggled to break the habit.

The disreputable practices typical in advertising products like Ryno's Remedy allowed the ethical industry, in later years, to lay most of the blame for the overuse of cocaine at the feet of the patent medicine business. Progressive Era reformers, eager for the cooperation of the ethical firms in crafting an apparatus of drug regulation, largely accepted this interpretation. As a consequence, reformers sometimes overlooked the ways in which both branches of the drug business had helped to develop a market for cocaine which was only marginally dependent on medical practice.

Cocaine appeared with the dawn of the modern pharmaceutical business, and the successful production and marketing of the drug served as an object lesson in the potential power of an enormous industrial enterprise. Largely ignoring physician claims to authority over the ways in which cocaine might be sold and used, drug makers marketed it aggressively beyond the informal limits of standard medical practice. Distinctions between ethical firms and patent medicine makers obscure the more fundamental commitment, shared by George S. Davis and Nathan S. Tucker, to influence national drug-taking habits.

Where careful distinctions are more useful is in sorting out the diverse products that shared coca or cocaine as an ingredient. These products were not simply vehicles for cocaine; indeed, in some instances, remedies traded upon the reputation of the drug without actually including cocaine as an ingredient. Rather, cocaine products fit into larger therapeutic categories, with a variety that defies simple characterization. Consumers and manufacturers alike understood that

Sutliff's Beef, Wine, and Coca was not easily interchangeable with Birney's Catarrh Cure or with Parke, Davis Voice Tablets. Moreover, the distinction between coca and cocaine, already carefully developed in the medical profession, carried over into the drug business. In the following years, however, all of these products would be swept away by an anticocaine crusade that cared little for such distinctions.

FIVE

The Transformation of Cocaine Use

The Popular Era, 1895–1920

In 1898, after nearly fifteen years of experience with cocaine in the United States, medical overuse of the drug remained central to perceptions of the national cocaine problem. In "The Abuse and Dangers of Cocaine," published that year, the *Medical News* concluded that the cocaine habit "in the majority of cases . . . results from the ill-advised prescription of the physician." The writer concluded that the medical community, in responding to instances of cocaine abuse, should not "go to the extreme in condemning it in its entirety." Careful voluntary controls seemed to be the answer: "cocain should never be placed in the hands of the patient under any circumstances, as the habit is so easily acquired. In this manner we may retain the use of a valuable drug and, by exercising proper care, eliminate its evil effects."[1] This cautious position, rather than a laissez faire credo, had been characteristic of the medical response since shortly after the introduction of cocaine into therapeutic practice.

The report, however, hinted at new patterns of use, including the popularity of cocaine sniffing in New Orleans. This was "not in the manner generally prescribed," for cocaine to be taken "not on account of its contractile effects on the nasal mucosa . . . but on account of its exhilarating effects."[2] Although Thomas Crothers still characterized the typical cocaine abuser in 1898 as a male professional older than thirty—the exact profile of the medical-era habitué—he also saw changes, reporting that "persons of the tramp and low criminal classes who use this drug are increasing in many of the cities. The cheapness and ease with which the drug can be obtained and the relief of pain and discomfort which follows its use make it very popular among this class."[3]

These and similar accounts document an increasing, though imperfect, awareness of the changing dimensions of the place of cocaine in American society. By 1903, despite the decline of medical interest in cocaine for therapeutic purposes (and active opposition by organized medicine to its largely unregulated distribution), the level of cocaine consumption in the United States had grown to about five times that of 1890. Nonmedical uses accounted for nearly the entire increase. In the process, the image of cocaine as an exclusive drug for "brain workers" gave way to the image of cocaine as the common man's drug, associated with laborers, youths, blacks, and the urban underworld.

Cocaine Sniffing and the Workplace

The popularization of cocaine began with its use by laborers as a stimulant. This pattern was not new; for centuries Latin American coca chewers relied upon the stimulant effect of the coca leaf to aid hard labor. In the nineteenth century, coca grown in Bolivia and Peru had found its way to agricultural laborers, mine workers, and other laboring groups that had long and difficult work requirements. As the noted eclectic physician John Uri Lloyd recalled regarding coca, "it was accepted by observing travelers that the leaves, being chewed, would yield an abundance of 'vital strength.'"[4]

Just where the use of cocaine for this purpose began in the United States is unclear. Early medical practice undoubtedly contributed to the popularization of cocaine as a stimulant. Physicians, of course, had employed cocaine most often as a *mental* stimulant; in the words of a Boston physician, it "renews the vigor of the intellect and relieves mental exhaustion, rendering the flow of thought more easy and the reasoning power more vigorous."[5] Many physicians and their patients, however, took note of its apparent utility in aiding physical endurance and strength as well.

The use of cocaine to sustain hard labor began among the roustabouts of New Orleans and the Mississippi River. These people occupied the bottom of the waterfront worker hierarchy, enduring long shifts of uninterrupted labor in handling ship cargoes. They earned a reputation for the "crushing labor" they performed and the "rollicking life" they led. At some point (probably around 1890), the roustabouts adopted cocaine as a drug compatible with the demands of hard labor and fast living.[6]

Most of the roustabouts were black, and to outside observers the blacks' use of cocaine seemed to confirm the racial stereotypes they already held. Medical opinion, shared by most employers, held that black workers were not only better able to endure physical labor but to endure environmental conditions that white workers could not. Cocaine supposedly increased these advantages, adding strength, endurance, and (according to the *Medical News*) making the black user "impervious to the extremes of heat and cold."[7]

Cocaine held obvious attractions for laborers. Opiates offered pain relief or escape but lacked the stimulant effects of cocaine. Cocaine sometimes replaced the work camp whisky ration for the same reason. Workers sniffed cocaine powders almost exclusively; cocaine powder was compact, transported easily, and used readily in workplace settings. Wherever large groups of workers engaged in intense physical labor, cocaine appeared. Writing in 1906, a Louisville physician declaring cocaine to be "alarmingly prevalent," traced much of its use to workers loading and unloading steamboats along the Mississippi.[8] Because waterfront employment was seasonal, roustabouts in search of work spread the use of cocaine throughout southern workplaces.[9] Harris Dickson, a lawyer living in Vicksburg, Mississippi, wrote that "the use of cocaine amongst the lower order of working negroes is quite common . . . It is common knowledge . . . throughout the country that on many public works, levee construction, railroad work and places of that sort where negroes congregate, that cocaine is handled by some method or other."[10]

Cocaine held attractions for employers as well. Many saw the drug as a means of increasing production and manipulating their workforce. Levee construction camps operating along the Mississippi River reportedly supplied cocaine to workers, as did many southern road construction camps. Mississippi River plantations also drew attention for distributing cocaine to agricultural laborers (who were increasingly in short supply in the region).[11] The *Medical News* reported that "one big planter is reported to keep the drug in stock among the plantation supplies and to issue regular rations of cocaine just as he was accustomed in the past to issue rations of whisky . . . As there is never enough labor to pick all the cotton it is to the interest of the planters to have the negroes work as much extra time as possible."[12] The same report claimed that "on many Yazoo plantations this year the negroes refused to work unless they could be assured that there was some place in the neighborhood where they could get cocaine." Rural counties in the heart of the Mississippi and Yazoo River plantation districts became focal points for charges and countercharges regarding cocaine distribution.[13]

In the West, mine employers and workers adopted cocaine in ways that paralleled the New Orleans experience. As early as August 1894, an Ohio physician reported that "in some portions of the West, especially in the mining regions, the use of cocaine, or 'cock,' as it is there called, as a stimulant is becoming very common."[14] Historian Henry Whiteside observed that in the 1890s, "cocaine was sold in the commissaries of many Colorado mining camps, but the white crystals quickly acquired a reputation for inciting violence and insanity." Moreover, the first state bill to control cocaine sales (in 1897) was introduced from La Plata County, a "center of mining activity."[15]

Cocaine appeared in the industrial Northeast at about the same time. Textile mills were particularly likely to have cocaine introduced by workers, supervisors, or employers. In Manchester, Connecticut, the home of many silk mills, one employer attempted to ease problems caused by irritating dust from the production process by supplying workers with a menthol and cocaine spray, to be taken on the job. In Maine, operatives from the textile mills in Lewiston purchased cocaine for their workers.[16] Nor was the use of cocaine limited to the textile industry. One druggist in Pittsburgh admitted "that he sold 40 to 50 oz. [of cocaine] a month, that engineers on one of the roads entering the city were getting to use it, because it kept them awake when working overtime."[17]

Was on-the-job cocaine use merely a tool of employers to increase production and worker dependence or an employee-driven initiative to enhance endurance and income?[18] The historical evidence remains inconclusive. Certainly some company stores stocked the drug, purchasing cocaine directly from wholesale drug houses (selling to retailers other than druggists was far more common in the South, which had both fewer druggists and fewer restrictions on the retailing of drug products). According to Harris Dickson, "cocaine is not 'forced upon negroes.' Contractors defend themselves by saying that if they do not furnish it somebody else will and their labor will leave them — likewise the profit."[19] Radical labor organizer "Big Bill" Haywood was not as sympathetic to the contractor. As a young man, Haywood traveled the mining regions of the West, where cocaine use flourished. He later observed that "at every company store, cocaine, morphine and heroin are sold. The workers, once addicted, cannot think of going away from their source of supply."[20]

Cocaine in the Underworld

Cocaine sniffing soon went from the work camp and factory to the urban vice district, where cocaine taking began to assume a more definite "deviant" identity. The earliest reports citing full-fledged cocaine "epidemics" arose from southern cities, with New Orleans leading the way in the 1890s. Newspaper accounts there noted the prominence of cocaine among the dance halls and saloons of Franklin Street. There, cocaine linked the dockworkers with the city's less-reputable neighborhoods because the roustabouts spent much of their free time on Franklin Street. Cocaine also appeared throughout the city's famous red-light district, Storyville, where "by 1900 cocaine had become by far the most common hard drug taken by poorer blacks and the prostitutes, black and white."[21] The city passed an ordinance against the sale of the drug, with the police chief reporting to his commanders that "the constant use of cocaine has assumed large and serious proportions and is daily increasing to such an extent as to be a menace to the public health." A grand jury concluded that "there are thousands of cocaine fiends in the city of New Orleans [the police estimate was a highly improbable 15,000 to 25,000, or roughly 4.5 to 7 percent of the city's population!] and that this habit, far from abating, is constantly growing."[22]

The earliest reporting of popular cocaine use appeared in a letter to the editors of the *American Druggist* concerning cocaine use in Dallas, Texas, in 1894. A growing city of about forty thousand residents, Dallas experienced an unprecedented rise in cocaine use, according to the obviously agitated correspondent, who observed that there were as many as six hundred people, "who had better be in their graves," suffering from the cocaine habit. Claiming the consumption of cocaine in Texas to have "increased fully ten-fold in the last two years," he warned of a spreading habit "incomparably more dangerous than the liquor habit." The Dallas report, although indicating a much lower prevalence of cocaine use than the New Orleans grand jury, did so in a near-hysterical tone that stressed two themes that would recur time and again: that the use of cocaine embodied a social threat far beyond simple health effects and that the drug held a special appeal among blacks and in "the lower quarters of the city."[23]

Anxiety-riddled reports detailing similar conditions appeared in cities throughout the South. The *American Druggist* informed its national readership that "it is no longer denied that the cocaine and morphine habits have spread to an alarming extent in some of the larger cities of the South" and used Chattanooga, Tennessee, to illustrate the "disastrous use of cocaine among the negroes and lower whites."[24] In 1900, state legislatures in Alabama, Georgia, and Tennessee considered anticocaine bills for the first time.[25] Although southern commentators decried the growing popularity of cocaine among underworld figures of both races, the assumption that blacks used the drug to a far greater extent than whites proved to be the source of the most intense anticocaine feeling. Although some observers claimed, as a New Orleans police officer did, that the use of cocaine "has always been confined to the immoral and lower classes of the community, both white and black," many others agreed with E. H. Williams' assertion that "the cocain habit has assumed the proportions of an epidemic among the colored people."[26]

The hostile response to the emergence of cocaine use among southern blacks reflected the supercharged racial tensions of the 1890s. The exhilarating effects of cocaine threatened to shatter carefully maintained social restraints; a movement to restrict alcohol had been under way since the Reconstruction Era for much the same reason, and cocaine seemed even more threatening. Whites perceived cocaine taking also as the manifestation of a newer, bolder attitude on the part of a "new generation" of young, urban blacks.[27] The *Atlanta Constitution* complained that "negroes can be seen at any time on the streets or in the Police Court snuffing the white powder."[28] Finally, the cocaine phenomenon seemed to confirm for whites (or could be used as a way of confirming) imagined black retrogression.[29] The effects of the drug were often described as transforming otherwise law-abiding blacks into beasts. A Houston druggist lectured his northern counterparts on the evils of cocaine addiction, finding a kind of moral lesson in the drug's popularity: "little did the North know, when freeing the negro, into what awful slavery they would lead him."[30]

The blatantly racist implications of these turn-of-the-century reports dictate that their core assumption be treated with great skepticism. The extent to which blacks were actually overrepresented in the cocaine-using population, however, is still an open question. Many historians dismiss the idea of cocaine popularity among black southerners out of hand, suggesting that "blacks probably used cocaine, like other prescription drugs, less than whites, simply because they had less money and less access to physicians" and that the "special association of cocaine with blacks, unlike the association of opium with Orientals, was probably baseless."[31] Yet cocaine *was* widely available in inexpensive forms such as catarrh cures or heavily adulterated snuffs, and distribution was very nearly independent of physicians by the late 1890s, so the lack of access to doctors was not a critical factor.

Still other elements of cocaine history indicate some basis for further exploration of the asserted connection between cocaine and blacks.[32] The popularity of cocaine in workplace settings dominated by black laborers, often promoted by employers, suggests one way in which the generalized use of cocaine could have begun in black communities. Moreover, enforcement of local alcohol prohibition laws in the South may have been particularly vigilant for blacks, making cocaine potentially more accessible than alcohol, at least initially. Finally, although the connection between cocaine and blacks may not be similar to the cultural connection between opium smoking and Chinese, in both instances urban residential neighborhoods were geographically part of, or adjacent to, areas where a great deal of drug distribution occurred. Thus, the geographical proximity of drug selling might explain both the perception and reality of cocaine use by nearby residents.[33]

In the remainder of the country, the association of cocaine and the residents of urban vice districts developed rapidly, leading one commentator to observe that "cocaine's reputation at present is more than shady . . . in every slum it is the favorite 'dope'; it leads men and women, boys and girls, into the stews, and it keeps them there."[34] New York City's tenderloin, Chicago's levee district, Pittsburgh's "Cocaine Street," and Kansas City's tenderloin all became centers of cocaine use and distribution (Figure 5.1). In an era of tightly segregated vice districts, it seemed natural that where other vices flourished, cocaine would as well.

Apart from the racial dimension of the cocaine underground, critics paid the greatest attention to the youthful users of the drug, citing its attractiveness to the young as a powerful illustration of its dangers. Without question, cocaine users were drawn increasingly from younger groups than previously; where some saw death and degeneracy, many young users found a marvelous escape along with feelings of well-being, power, and strength. Jessie Binford, a resident of Hull House specializing in juvenile delinquency (later head of the Chicago Juvenile Protective Association), suggested that "cocaine is far more tempting than morphine to the young and healthy." Many reported feelings of strength and importance or felt as if they were some notable figure of fame or wealth. Inmates of Pittsburgh's Western Penitentiary claimed that "it [cocaine] makes us feel like millionaires."[35] Dr. Alice Hamilton, Hull House resident and public health reformer, recalled in her memoirs that "the boys told us they felt delightfully queer, 'as if I was going up in a flying machine, as if I was a millionaire and could do anything I pleased.'"[36]

The sale of "this death-dealing drug" to "children," as one account termed it, was the subject of much comment and concern. Images of young children being preyed upon in schoolyards were particularly common. *Hampton's Magazine* suggested that in Newark, New Jersey, children as young as eight had used the drug, and Harvey Wiley reported in *Good Housekeeping* sales of cocaine to schoolchildren by "sweets vendors."[37] Despite the popularity of such claims, there is little evidence that young children used cocaine to any extent.[38]

It was not uncommon, however, for a report on cocaine use among children actually to be referring to sixteen- or eighteen-year-olds. These users were almost exclusively males. A Des Moines newspaper, complaining of teenage boys wandering around in "dopy glee," was merely one reflection of a more widespread reaction against these young recreational users. Another description claimed that "the cocaine habit is steadily growing in Newark among the boys who play pool in the upstairs pool and billiard rooms and that the usual way of taking the powder is by snuffing it up the nostrils from a quill." Worse, the report continued, "the assertion is made that scores of young men have recently lost ambition and em-

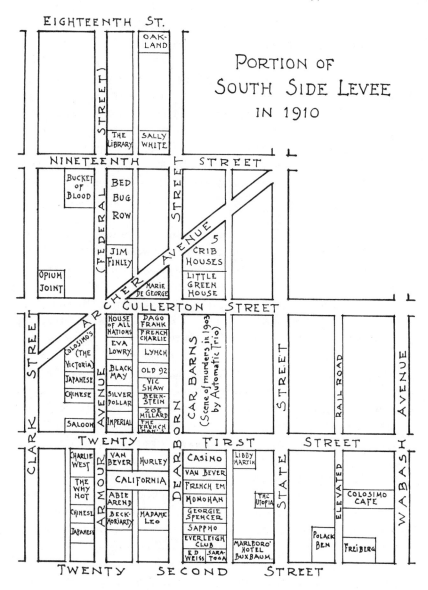

Figure 5.1 Chicago levee district. Herbert Asbury's popular work *Gem of the Prairie* told the story of the Chicago underworld. This map, reproduced in that work, illustrates a portion of the city's levee district. Most of the locations identified were houses of prostitution, but this district also housed most of the Chicago cocaine sellers. The car barns in the center of the map were the scene of a notorious rampage by the youths (known as the "Car Barn Bandits" and the "Automatic Trio") widely rumored to have been cocaine fiends.

ployment by the use of the drug in this manner and that several deaths have recently been caused by the habit."[39]

Whereas cocaine threatened young men, the close identification of cocaine with prostitutes embodied multiple threats. Some suggested that cocaine was a lure to prostitution, an idea often linked to the Progressive Era crusade against "white slavery." The fight against prostitution emphasized the victimization of young women, enticed or forced to prostitute themselves by predatory white slavers. Entrapping women with a ready supply of drugs seemed to be an obvious way in which agents might, as one journalist described, "cunningly persuade young girls who have fallen into their power to take up cocaine. 'Have a sniff of this; it won't hurt you, and it will cheer you up,' they say; and then the unhappy creature loses all desire to escape."[40]

If cocaine seemed to be a means by which young women might be led to moral ruin, the cocaine-sniffing prostitute became the means by which the habit of drug taking might be spread to others. The world of "the lower class of prostitutes and their followers and the similar class of criminals," in the words of a New York City police officer in the tenderloin district, became a center of moral contagion, a description not unlike that used to explain the venereal disease problem.[41] The moral contagion model offered an easily understood explanation for the spread of cocaine use, and the influence of the model on popular thought revealed itself in sources as diverse as a 1903 American Pharmaceutical Association (APhA) report describing "two cases of men who acquired the cocaine habit from lewd women they visited habitually," and the claim of New York City Police Commissioner Bingham that "the classes of the community most addicted to the habitual use of cocaine are the parasites who live on the earnings of prostitutes, prostitutes of the lowest order, and young degenerates who acquire the habit through their connection with prostitutes or parasites."[42]

Cocaine powders and catarrh cures emerged quickly as the principal "underworld" forms of cocaine, "rapidly supplanting in part the use of morphine" according to more than one report. Cocaine snuffs were "a conveniently portable and easily used form," according to the APhA, "sold in large quantities to a certain class of men and women — the 'powers that prey' — under the name of 'Brighteye,' from the effect of the drug in giving the eyes a temporary brilliancy."[43] On New York's Lower East Side, cocaine takers employed snuffing bottles (often purchased with catarrh cures): " 'Snuffing' is done by the use of a bottle having two glass tubes passing through the cork. 'Catarrh powder' or other mixtures are placed in the bottle and the snuffer blows down on one tube, placing the other in his nose."[44] The ease with which the powders could be bought and used, combined with the other temptations of city vice districts, led one popular magazine to warn readers that "even if, so far, it has flourished principally among already depraved elements in the big cities, it is well not to forget the contagious character of all vice."[45]

Cocaine and Opiates

In cities of the Northeast and West, the emergence of cocaine use also corresponded to an apparent decline in the popularity of opium smoking, which had been the most popular underworld form of drug taking. Opium smoking appeared in the Chinatowns and tenderloins (these areas were often contiguous) of cities across the country, attracting many non-Chinese recreational users.

The tenderloin district of Philadelphia was one of many to experience the transition from opium smoking to cocaine sniffing. Within the tenderloin lay the city's Chinatown, a center for opium smoking and opium selling in the 1870s and 1880s. For a time, fashionable theatergoers concluded their evenings at nearby opium-smoking establishments, but by the first decade of the twentieth century, cocaine sniffing had replaced opium smoking as the leading recreational drug habit. Reverend Frederic Poole, head of the Christian League Chinatown Mission, noted in 1909 that white opium smokers appeared to "yield still further to that other and still more harmful habit, the use of Cocaine."[46] Philadelphia physician S. Solis Cohen suggested that "among the vicious classes cocaine is, I believe, driving out opium."[47]

A druggist who spent several months working in a pharmacy in the Philadelphia tenderloin observed the growing importance of cocaine to the drug culture of the community. In a neighborhood where "the number of men and women, in the prime of life, addicted to the laudanum, paregoric, morphine and cocaine is appalling," the druggist reported that "cocaine, of which the muriate is generally sold, is dispensed in crystals and also in solution, as ordered by the customer, and is used by the fiend by mouth and hypodermically." The catarrh snuff predominated; "the buyers of this article, being acquainted with the nature of it, buy it to get the desired effect."[48]

Opium smoking did not, of course, immediately disappear in Philadelphia. Many opium smokers continued to use their drug (particularly in Chinatown), but cocaine was now an equally visible presence. A young man who arrived in the Philadelphia tenderloin in about 1907 was struck by the ubiquity of drug use among his neighbors. Employed as a clerk and houseman in a hotel near 9th and Race Streets, "in the heart of Philadelphia's Chinatown," the young man lived alongside numerous vice district characters, including Chinatown Whitie, Butch Turner, Two Bits, Peanuts, Blonde May, Chinatown Mae, the Girl in Blue, and

Ann Nolan, "all of them notorious and known to half the men in the U.S. Navy and Marine Corps — all of them users of opium or its derivatives." At the hotel, "one could smoke for twenty-five cents. Morphine, heroin, and cocaine could be had for fifty and sixty cents per dram."[49]

One inducement away from smoking opium was the increasing pressure on smokers from law enforcement. Although opium smoking had been tolerated to varying degrees, by the 1890s efforts to control its use were under way in many major cities. Such efforts were aided by the relatively high profile of opium smokers; most use took place in opium "dens" well known to police, and the smoking itself was easy to detect because of the drug's powerful odor. Cocaine, on the other hand, presented far fewer risks. As the San Diego chief of police observed, "Cocaine snuffing is taking the place of opium smoking here, as the dope fiends find it much more convenient to use, and the chances of detection less, the use of cocaine is increasing rapidly."[50]

Although cocaine sniffing supplanted opium smoking among underworld users, cocaine in combination with morphine (and later, heroin) added an entirely new dimension. Intravenous morphine users turned to cocaine and found the combination of the two drugs irresistible, a circumstance first acknowledged in the medical era. Used either in alternating or combined doses, the pairing increased steadily in popularity among nonmedical users. In contrast to the cocaine sniffers, combination opiate/cocaine users most frequently injected the drug because that was the most typical route of administration for morphine.

An early attempt to characterize drug use emphasized the relationship between cocaine and the opiates among "drug fiends": "They commence with smoking opium, which becomes too expensive and consumes too much time, so they eat morphine; then they use it by injection, because it goes further; then they tip their injection off with cocaine, because it deadens the pain, and gradually they use more cocaine than morphine."[51] Although this description overlooks individual variation, opiate/cocaine users appeared in significant number in addict populations, where they had not been previously. An 1899 survey of one thousand drug patients, all of whom applied for treatment at the Keeley Institute in Dwight, Illinois, before 1897, reveals that the institution was already treating many multiple-drug users. According to the report, 59 addicts used opium, 751 used morphine, 166 used combinations of opiates and cocaine, whereas only 18 used cocaine alone.[52]

By 1919, even as the overall levels of cocaine consumption in the United States declined, surveys of drug addicts showed that opiate/cocaine users were still around. The first 3,262 patients treated at the Worth Street narcotic clinic in New

TABLE 5.1
Number of Narcotic Clinic Patients Categorized
by Drug of Addiction

Drug	No. of Patients
Cocaine	6
Cocaine and morphine	42
Cocaine and heroin	305
Morphine	690
Morphine and heroin	41
Heroin	2,178

SOURCE: Data from the New York City narcotic clinic are cited in Hans W. Maier, *Der Kokainismus,* trans. Oriana Josseau Kalant (Toronto: Addiction Research Foundation, 1987).

York City in 1919 were categorized by drug of addiction (Table 5.1). Although the percentage of addicts using cocaine (12%) was lower than the 18 percent of Keeley patients, reflecting the spread of heroin in postwar New York City, combination use persisted more notably than exclusive cocaine use.[53] Combination drug use gradually acquired an association with the underground drug environment. The percentage of cocaine/morphine users was often considerably higher, for example, in institutions whose addicts came largely from the underground population. Surveys of addicts in city hospitals and prisons indicated that as many as one quarter or more of all addicts injected cocaine in combination with morphine.[54]

The trend among drug users was not exclusively opiate use followed by the addition of cocaine. Some cocaine users certainly learned to balance some of the undesirable effects of the cocaine with either alcohol or morphine. The introduction of heroin (the drug that eventually would largely replace cocaine among underworld drug users) in 1898 reinforced and accelerated the trend toward multiple drug use among those whose initial drug had been cocaine.[55]

Readily available in the first decade after its introduction, heroin could either be sniffed or injected, so that cocaine users of all kinds could easily turn to it. A 1913 editorial in the *American Druggist* warned its readers that "a new danger has arisen" concerning heroin, reporting that "in Pennsylvania there is no restriction on its sale at present, and unfortunate cocaine victims have turned to it as an easily obtained substitute for the more deadly drug they have come to depend on as a necessity of life." The editorial noted that "heroin is used by them just as cocaine was, that is, as a snuff, inhaling the powdered drug up the nostrils being the most general method."[56]

In sum, cocaine use in the late nineteenth century conformed to no simple pattern. Aficionados had complicated drug-using careers, like that of "Dawson Sue," a San Francisco drug addict. Asked how she started on "the habit," she responded:

A man broke me in. I started on the pipe — smoking opium. It was great fun at first, and then one morning I woke up and realized that it was no longer play — that it was a habit. Then the law knocked over smoking and I took to heroin. I sniffed it and in 3 minutes I had the "kick" that opium took 2 and 3 hours to give me. A lot of us didn't know really what heroin — sniff H — was, until after it was too late. And then the reaction was terrible. It takes your memory you know. After a while you can't think. I got scared and quit and took up cocaine and morphine. I guess that's just as bad, though.[57]

The Transformation of the Cocaine User

The middle-aged professionals who dominated the medical era had been overshadowed by newer groups. The only consistency between the medical and popular eras was the dominance of males in surveys of users. This was particularly true for popular-era habitués housed in public hospitals and jails, where young males were already overrepresented. A survey of addicts received at the workhouse on Blackwell's Island in New York City indicated that 90.5 percent were male, whereas a Philadelphia General Hospital survey reported that 70.1 percent of all cases were male. Many had initiated use between the ages of sixteen and twenty-five.[58]

By this time, the origins of cocaine use were much less likely to involve any medical treatment. A 1916 study of 147 drug patients from the Philadelphia General Hospital indicated that three quarters of cocaine addicts were more likely than other addicts to have begun the use of the drug through personal associations or for social reasons and outside of medical care (see Table 5.2). The authors concluded that "while these surveys prove conclusively that a vast majority of cases of opium smoking, heroin, and cocaine sniffing are acquired through association, we would emphasize the fact that the largest single factor in the production of morphinism has been professional medication."[59] Other early-twentieth-century surveys of drug addicts suggested approximately the same distribution.[60] As a journalist observed, "one cocaine fiend will induce a friend to try his pet dissipation, and so the habit spreads, in a kind of endless chain . . . they are a strange, uncanny tribe, these 'coke' fiends."[61]

In his 1915 report, "The Number and Kind of Drug Addicts," Martin Wilbert

TABLE 5.2
Origins of Addiction, Philadelphia General Hospital Study

Origins of Use	Morphine Addicts	Heroin Addicts	Cocaine Addicts
Physicians	33	0	0
Substitute for opium smoking	20	20	0
Substitute for heroin	6	0	0
Association/social	18	56	32
Self-medication	10	0	1
Relieve effect of other drugs	0	7	10
TOTAL	87	83	43

SOURCE: Joseph McIver and George E. Price, *JAMA* 66 (1916): 476–80.

concluded that "practically all authorities are agreed that the continued use of cocaine is a vice rather than a disease," whereas addiction to opium and morphine "is generally recognized as a condition over which the individual patient has little or no control."[62] Wilbert's definition of cocaine use as a vice derived partly from the view that cocaine, unlike morphine, was not physically addicting and was therefore only a habit. Yet the origins of use also shaped the medical and social views of the user. Opiate addicts, for example, had always been placed in a separate category from those addicted to opium smoking. A Wisconsin physician developed a three-part classification system for morphine and cocaine addicts based solely on the origins of their use: first, "those who acquired the drug habit because of chronic painful ailments"; second, "those who resorted to drugs because of acute and perhaps relapsing ailments"; and finally, "those who, although free from physical ailments resort to the use of morphin in order to free themselves of painful psychic disturbances as mental depression and insomnia, also those who acquire its use in search of new sensations." The author noted that users in this third group were those "who rush to gratify every desire . . . heedless of the future evil which may be resultant upon so doing."[63]

Such distinctions were accepted widely among public health and law enforcement officials. In 1923, W. C. Fowler, health officer of the District of Columbia and a practicing physician for thirty-five years, analyzed the use of the term *dope fiend.* Not all addicts, he felt, could properly be called *fiends,* because many were "high-grade citizens, persons who occupy high positions, both socially and economically." The term, Fowler wrote, was best reserved for those underworld persons "who were originally mentally and morally degenerates" and who began their use "through a desire to gratify certain sensual pleasure."[64]

This increasingly common association of cocaine use with social settings and pleasure seeking contributed, in three related ways, to the negative perception of users. First, it appeared to confirm that cocaine users, by using the drug for pleasure, were purposefully establishing a deviant identity.[65] Cocaine sniffing on the job to increase endurance could claim a tenuous connection to the therapeutic application of the drug. Recreational use, emphasizing the euphoric and mood-altering effects of cocaine, broke the connection to "legitimate" consumption entirely. Consequently, cocaine sniffing (like opium smoking) became a vice, rather than a necessity, earning only condemnation.

Second, nonmedical use of cocaine removed the blame from the shoulders of the physicians. Problems associated with cocaine were solely the fault of the user. The dramatic expansion of nonmedical consumption transformed the medical wonder drug into a social vice. These changes, in both use and perception, occurred *before,* not after, prohibition. Drug prohibition merely built upon a set of negative images already well developed.

Third, the social settings of cocaine consumption led authorities to liken cocaine users to carriers of a contagious disease, and in much the same way that a disease carrier required removal to quarantine, the need to protect the general public justified strict control of cocaine users.[66] A New York City physician observed that the public had considerable sympathy for "the innocent and ignorant formation" of drug habits but that "the vicious user of a drug whose sole excuse is the seeking for new sensations, is a person who does not need protection, but rather restraint by law in order that he may not become a menace to the public weal and a care for the public charities."[67] The aggressive public response to the growth of popular cocaine consumption contradicts the contention by several historians that a laissez faire attitude characterized public policy toward cocaine in the preprohibition era.

SIX

Private Acts, Public Concerns
The Emergence of the Cocaine Fiend

A cocaine user, a recent prisoner in a Chicago police station, described his experiences with the drug to a reporter from the Chicago *Record-Herald* in autumn 1908.

> I was floating on a soft cloud that moved through a glowing paradise. The floors were of gold and the windows of rubies. Ivory bushes sprouted leaves of delicate silver; a million birds filled the air with their music; servants ran around with trays of food and drink; marble fountains tinkled with sweet sounds. The air was filled with the perfume of violets; diamond dust hung over me — and then a policeman arrested me.[1]

The startling contrasts of the account, even allowing for some license on the part of the reporter, highlight the entanglements of preprohibition drug users with state authority.

That certain persons might need to fear the approach of a policeman in the midst of their drug-inspired visions and ecstasies is not immediately obvious in retrospect. Most middle-class opiate users in the nineteenth century successfully kept years (and even lifetimes) of drug consumption and addiction private. Nor was there much in the way of formal legislation to suggest that the public was greatly concerned about regulating the behavior of these opiate addicts. Their situation and the presumed right to private drug consumption have led some scholars to characterize this period as a "dope fiend's paradise."[2]

To the extent that the advent of national drug prohibition, with the passage of the Harrison Act in 1914, forced nearly every opiate addict and cocaine user outside the law, this earlier era *was* a legal paradise for some. What this characterization obscures, however, are the efforts by state and local government to restrict certain kinds of drug use. These interventions focused state attention on the "pleasure users" of cocaine, whose disturbing presence produced a new descriptive term, the *cocaine fiend*. Rarely the result of formal legal controls on drug use or possession, state action typically evolved as a response to two sets of concerns: cocaine use as an endangerment to the public health, and the socially aberrant behavior of users as a threat to public safety.

Anxiety-filled reports describing the damaging effects of cocaine circulated widely around the turn of the century. For those with the necessary resources, private treatment facilities and asylums were available when the physical or social costs of a cocaine habit grew intolerable. Those without resources, however, found precious little publicly funded treatment available when their own circumstances demanded positive intervention. Instead, the growing medical and popular perception that cocaine use was a degenerative vice, not a genuine "addiction," limited systematic public response markedly. Intervention was consequently less welcome and limited to short-term detention hospitals, to police drunk tanks for "sobering up," or to lengthy incarcerations in prisons and workhouses.

Chronic and heavy cocaine consumption took an obvious physical toll, but the popular literature focused on the central concern of public order. Here, in the pages of the nation's newspapers and magazines, negative attitudes ran well ahead of formal prohibitionist legislation. Connections among cocaine, crime, and vice were made often and very directly. Few doubted that cocaine users were, in the words of the *Record-Herald* reporter, "active roots of vice and degeneracy."[3] Although the drug underworld almost certainly overlapped with the criminal underworld to some extent, the most frightening product of this connection was also the most mythical: the cocaine-crazed violent predator whose very humanity had been destroyed by the drug. Few responses, however harsh, could not be justified by the threat this imagined fiend posed to communities.

"Habits of the Mind": Cocaine Use and Public Health

From the earliest years of medical use, most descriptions of cocaine counted the drug as among the most seductive of substances. Cocaine appeared to lack the unpleasant side effects of other drugs, including alcohol, which were thought to set natural limits on consumption. In the words of a Philadelphia physician, cocaine could be "the most insidious of all drug habits . . . use of the drug being unaccompanied by disagreeable after-effects."[4] In this manner, the physician concluded, "the vice is readily and rapidly established."

The most immediate source of public concern, however, had less to do with the ease of obtaining a cocaine habit or even the difficulty in effecting a cure, but rather with the so-called *coke drunks* whose public intoxication invited intervention. Their episodes included acute negative reactions to cocaine as well as various kinds of cocaine-inspired hallucinations and psychoses, the bizarre novelty of which added to the reputation of cocaine as a destructive drug. In 1898, the *Canada Lancet* published a remarkably detailed description of the physical progression of the cocaine abuser. In addition to the pallor, emaciation, and nervousness common to many abusers, the periodical described the paranoia and hallucinations as well as the "coke bugs": "an imaginary body which the patient believes to be real, usually assuming the form of minute worms and insects situated under the skin, so that he will mutilate his body, especially his hands and fingers, trying to dig them out with the point of a pen-knife or other suitable sharp-pointed instrument."[5]

Persons under the influence of cocaine found their way into city drunk tanks and police hospitals after the turn of the century. In the Philadelphia General Hospital drunk and detention wards, cocaine users accounted for 31.3 percent of all drug users receiving treatment between 1904 and 1906.[6] The worst cases, according to those who treated them, were hypodermic users of morphine and cocaine in combination. C. W. Boynge, an assistant police surgeon at the Los Angeles City Receiving Hospital, explained that "our City Jail is never free from the worst class — the user of the needle — and at times contains as high as twenty-five or thirty of these habitués . . . in a few of the cases mentioned as being habitués, the drug used was cocaine, but those using this drug alone were few. Many of them use it in conjunction with the opiates, however."[7]

The physical effects of long-term cocaine abuse were no less serious, particularly when compared with the experiences of opiate addicts. Many *opiate* addicts moved with relative ease through decades of addiction, able to manage their habits and remain functional. Perhaps most shocking were the visible signs of deterioration and dysfunction in long-term cocaine users, as described by physician N. S. Yawger: "rapid emaciation, the individual is distressed of countenance, is restless, talkative, and secretive, the skin has a pale, yellowish, withered appearance, the eyes are deeply sunken and the pupils dilated."[8]

Physical and mental distress among cocaine users were not substantially a product of social or economic standing nor a mere creation of biased observers because some of the therapeutically addicted physicians and professionals of the 1880s had displayed virtually identical breakdowns during the medical era. The popularization of cocaine, however, brought these agonies more directly to the attention of local governments. The criminal justice system had the most immediate contact with this new group of problem users. In a typical scene, five cocaine users arrested during raids on drug sellers writhed and begged for cocaine while awaiting arraignment in a New York City courthouse. As a newspaper account described it, "as the hour set for the hearing drew near yesterday it was seen that the five prisoners were in no condition to be taken before the Magistrate. The men could scarcely stand alone." Not knowing what other course to take, a health inspector ordered that the five be given some cocaine to get them through their hearings.[9]

With the accumulation of experience came calls for a more systematic public response. In early 1907, the *New York Times* reported a warning from the chief of the psychopathic ward at Bellevue Hospital that "unless something was done to put a stop to the manner in which some druggists sold cocaine, the hospitals would soon be filled with cocaine users." Indeed, the newspaper reported that many local hospitals already had a "cocaine ward set aside especially for the treatment of cocaine fiends."[10] The fiends in these places were generally given short-term detention and treatment, usually consisting of detoxification only. On the surface, the detoxification regimen appeared to be particularly appropriate for cocaine abusers. Without the difficult physical withdrawal process experienced by opiate addicts, most cocaine abusers seemed to sober up quickly and return to normal. Reliance on short-term detention reflected an absence of public institutions for the long-term custody of cocaine fiends, leaving jail as the easiest place for sobering up. A Chicago report complained that "aside from the Bridewell, there is no hospital or dispensary in the city where free treatment for the cocaine habit can be had and no place where such treatment can be had at a price within the means of the average person indulging in the habit."[11]

The experience of George Wilson, a forty-one-year-old homeless resident of Syracuse, New York, shows the extremes of the physical impact of cocaine as well as the typical method of dealing with the cocaine fiend. In June 1906, Wilson was discovered sprawled out on the bank of a canal. When the Syracuse police and health bureau found him, he was unconscious and holding a hypodermic needle in one hand and a bottle in the other. According to the *Syracuse Herald,* officers took Wilson to the police station, "where frequent applications of the drug had to be administered to prevent his going into a delirium, the officers characterized the case as one of the most pitiable of a similar nature they had ever witnessed."[12]

Wilson's appearance in court the next day was scarcely better. The newspaper recorded that "he trembled like an aspen-leaf . . . his eyes were bulging from their sockets and he was wild looking." Health Inspector James Maloney explained to the justice that Wilson had begun using cocaine three years earlier and "that since then he had been a hopeless 'dope' fiend." Maloney also noted that Wilson had been sent to "the County house" once before but had returned without a cure for

TABLE 6.1
Massachusetts Drug Addicts by Drug of Addiction, 1917

Drug	Norfolk State Hospital	Private Physician	Totals
Morphine	70.3% (90)	30.2% (80)	43.3% (170)
Heroin	14.8% (19)	4.5% (12)	7.9% (31)
Opium	0.0% (0)	4.2% (11)	2.8% (11)
Multiple opiates	5.5% (7)	7.5% (20)	6.9% (27)
Cocaine	0.8% (1)	0.0% (0)	0.3% (1)
Cocaine and opiates	8.6% (11)	53.6% (142)	38.9% (153)
TOTAL	100% (128)	100% (265)	100.1% (393)

SOURCE: Massachusetts Legislature, *Report of the Commission to Investigate the Extent of the Use of Habit-Forming Drugs,* House Document 149 (Boston: January 1917), p. 10; reprint, *Public Policy and the Problem of Addiction,* ed. Gerald N. Grob (New York: Arno Press, 1981).

his addiction. By Wilson's own account, a physician had started him on the drug, which he desperately wished to discontinue. Wilson pleaded to the court, "I want to stop, my God, I want to stop!"[13] His purchase and possession of cocaine were, it should be emphasized, entirely legal. Nevertheless, authorities believed that his condition merited some kind of response. Inspector Maloney argued in police court that "this man is all gone and needs to be sent to an institution."[14] The judge sentenced the unfortunate addict to six months in the penitentiary, where "every effort will be made . . . to cure Wilson of the drug habit during his stay."[15]

Commitment to public asylums or long-term care facilities proved far less likely for cocaine users than for opiate addicts or alcoholics. This relative exclusion of cocaine habitués from public treatment institutions owed a great deal to the perception of cocaine as a potentially degenerative vice rather than as a drug that led to an addiction requiring intensive medical intervention. Turn-of-the-century commentators, however, had no shortage of additional explanations for why this was so. N. S. Yawger had spent several years treating nervous diseases at both the Philadelphia Hospital for the Insane and the drunk and detention wards of Philadelphia General Hospital and had observed that few cocaine users were ever transferred from the detention wards to the Hospital for the Insane. He explained that cocaine users "seldom become chronic insane patients but usually die in a marasmic (physical wasting) condition or are carried off" by some intervening illness.[16]

Whatever the cause, cocaine users were but a small minority in most treatment institutions. Table 6.1, for example, presents data on drug addicts in Massachusetts. Several observations regarding the Massachusetts data are pertinent. First, few cocaine addicts received treatment, except those using the drug in combination with morphine or heroin. Second, for these combination users, the difference in treatment setting was quite pronounced. More than half of the addicts being treated on an outpatient basis were users of opiates and cocaine, whereas fewer than one tenth of institutionalized drug addicts were combination users.

Finally, where physicians made sustained therapeutic efforts to cure the cocaine habit, their poor results further frustrated the expansion of treatment. On the one hand, cocaine users appeared to return to good health more rapidly and easily than opiate addicts and so were often released quickly. Many of these individuals, however, soon relapsed. Charles Collins, writing in the popular periodical *Everyday Life,* articulated the general sense of skepticism regarding successful treatment. Collins observed no "excruciating torment" suffered by users deprived of cocaine (the experience of George Wilson notwithstanding); indeed, one of "these people" locked up in prison for an extended period of time would seem to outgrow a need for the drug entirely. Still, Collins claimed, the inevitable result of sending such a person back to the city "as a free agent" and "a man with an apparently rehabilitated will" was a return to cocaine. Within twenty-four hours, "he is in the throes of a 'coke' debauch."[17]

Echoing Collins' pessimism, numerous personal accounts described an intense psychological craving for the drug which failed to cease with the withdrawal of cocaine and might persist for years. Jessie Binford of Hull House related the depressing case of a twenty-four-year-old cocaine abuser who applied to the settlement house for relief. She arranged to have the young man work on the distant farm of some friends. After having used the money provided for a railroad ticket to buy cocaine, he "hoboed" his way to the farm, where he worked for three years without cocaine use. At this point, the young man was allowed to return to Chicago, where after two hours he spent all of his savings. Binford finally discovered him in his police station cell.[18]

Some argued that the minimal treatment most cocaine users received contributed to treatment failures. Thomas Simonton thought that even two or three months might be too short a time in which to obtain useful results. Instead, he urged that six months to a year should be invested "to build these sufferers up and improve their general health so that they may be better prepared to resist the temptation to return to their old habits when set free." On the whole, however, most studies of the cocaine habit regarded successful intervention as problematic. Reports from long-term treatment facilities did little to suggest that cocaine addicts were curable under the best of circumstances. Simonton himself asked "how many really stay cured?" and concluded that "of all drugs, cocaine addiction is the hardest to break off."[19] In California, addicts could be committed to state hospitals for the insane for two to twelve months, during which time they were to be "restored to a normal condition." An official of a state board of pharmacy concluded that "it is sad to relate that the reports from these institutions show that 95 percent of those who are sent out as cured, return to the habit sooner or later."[20] Well before national prohibition, the medical and popular consensus anticipated the later observation of Arthur Woods that "no medical treatment can eradicate the habit patterns of the human mind."[21]

Law Enforcement and the Control of Cocaine Users

The expansion of nonmedical cocaine use, particularly among groups already regarded as socially marginal or threatening, raised serious concerns about the impact of the drug on social order. The novel stimulant and euphoriant effects of cocaine accounted for some of these concerns. The absence of specific legislation prohibiting cocaine use required local authorities to be inventive and develop a variety of indirect mechanisms to control consumption. By far the most typical strategy involved the application of nuisance laws pertaining to "vagrancy" and "disturbing the peace."[22]

Arrests of *sellers* for violations of cocaine-vending statutes frequently produced an even larger number of *customers* arrested for vagrancy. In the absence of restrictive legislation or supplementary legislation that focused exclusively on the regulation of sellers, police employed arrests on other charges to control underworld cocaine users. In Pittsburgh, police "endeavored to bolster rather lax laws," according to the chief, "by unremitting effort to break up the practice by the exploiter and the victim" (see Figure 6.1). This effort included arresting the "victims" and sending them to the county workhouse for short terms; "as many as 100 cocaine fiends have been arrested in one month . . . cocaine produced nearly as many court cases as alcohol."[23]

Chicago police conducted raids on thirty-five sites of cocaine sales during 1911 and 1912, netting about one hundred arrests, yet authorities held only nineteen of the arrestees for violations of state drug laws. The remainder "were booked under disorderly charges as inmates or prospective purchasers."[24] Several years earlier, a Chicago police officer had complained that drug addicts "should be properly cared for in institutions and not [subjected] to the inevitable results of being arrested under vagrancy or other laws governing disorderly conduct." Such a solution, the officer argued, would do much to "relieve Peace Officers of great responsibility of caring for individuals under the influence . . . over night in premises ill provided for their care."[25]

Other informal avenues were also available to control undesirable behavior stemming from drug use, especially among juveniles. Consider the case of sixteen-year-old George Fromme. George and his friends had begun to use cocaine by chipping in to purchase (legally) "catarrhal and toothache" prepara-

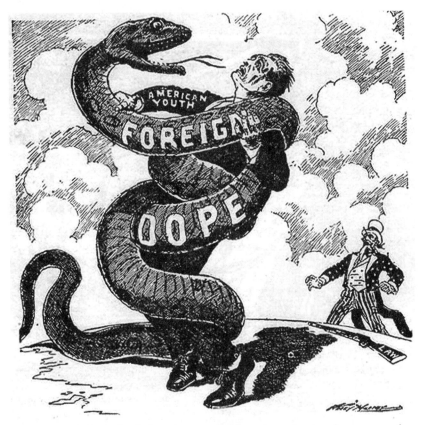

Figure 6.1. With the decline in American-produced cocaine and opiates by 1920, popular representations continued to use the traditional menacing images, but increasingly emphasized the "foreign" aspects of the drug problem. Here, a 1922 cartoon shows Uncle Sam's only defense, a rifle marked "law," lying on the ground. *Seattle Post-Intelligencer.*

tions from various drugstores. Eventually the boys found one druggist willing to sell them cocaine by the ounce (in violation of New York City and New York State law). According to his mother, George often came home "in a dazed condition" whereupon she was "compelled to roll him around the floor of her home . . . to straighten him out." At the time his story was reported, George was in the New York City Tombs, awaiting a hearing.[26] He had been arrested on a complaint from his mother after he sold a new suit of clothes at a pawnshop to buy cocaine.

The indirect legal devices by which local authorities dealt with underworld cocaine users suggest that official reports of drug arrests do not accurately reflect actual trends in law enforcement. In New York State, for example, after implementation of the so-called Boylan Law in 1914, the annual number of drug cases received in the New York City Court of Special Sessions increased from 106 to 1,415.[27] Although the new legislation almost certainly influenced law enforcement to a degree, there is good reason to believe that many of those arrested would have faced non–drug charges in earlier years. Similarly, drug arrests in New Orleans for 1911 totaled 70 but reached 316 in 1914, the first year in which arrests were made under the city's Poisonous Drug Act.[28]

Police efforts aimed at breaking up the cocaine trade proved to be another significant source of official harassment for cocaine consumers. Because possession of cocaine was not in itself a crime in many jurisdictions, police actually had to prove that a sale had taken place in order to make an arrest. The problem, as a San Francisco police sergeant observed, was that "the cocaine dealer has one great advantage from detection and arrest in selling this drug, owing to the fact that a cocaine fiend can be easily identified, thereby eliminating his chances of detection by a decoy."[29] The solution, then, was to coerce actual cocaine abusers into serving as buyers for the police. When Chicago police complained that they "were allowed no money with which to hire 'stools' or habitual users," a reform commission observed that "a cocaine 'fiend' under arrest under a vagrancy charge will gladly make the purchases for a little leniency."[30]

Reflecting this pattern of enforcement, cocaine users in custody tended to predominate in local jails and night courts rather than among the more serious offenders. Hamilton Wright, inquiring as to the percentage of criminals using cocaine in New York City, found that cocaine users comprised an estimated 5 percent of prisoners in the New York City Tombs, whereas officials "at the Jefferson Market Tenderloin station" suggested a much higher percentage, "mostly for trifling offenses, and who are quickly fined and discharged, and who rarely commit crimes that would lead them to the Tombs."[31] Charles B. Whilden, secretary of the California State Board of Pharmacy, made a similar observation: "of the criminals in the State Penitentiaries, about 7 percent only are 'dope fiends,' but a very much larger proportion of those sent to city Prisons and County Jails belong to this class, as few of the crimes committed by them are felonies, most of them are misdemeanors."[32]

Users involved in other vice trades were, of course, subject to considerable police supervision. Of all vice-related criminal activities, prostitution was perhaps most closely linked to cocaine use. Not surprisingly, then, prostitutes constituted a significant proportion of cocaine users under police custody or surveillance. A report from the Baltimore City jail offers one indication of this pattern of law enforcement activity. Of forty-seven drug-using prisoners, forty-three were women, "nearly all colored." Their average age was twenty-four, and most were surely prostitutes. Only six cases indicated medical addiction. More significantly, only five of the prisoners had been arrested for crimes committed to buy the drug. A breakdown of the prisoners by the drug used suggests the prominence of cocaine: nine morphine, seventeen cocaine, sixteen morphine and cocaine, two laudanum, two morphine and laudanum, and one all.[33]

A final source of police contact with cocaine users, of course, included criminal activity by users, unrelated to the drug use itself. The question of user criminality was, then as now, the subject of considerable debate and interest. During 1908 and 1909, while serving as a U.S. delegate to the Shanghai Opium Conference, Dr. Hamilton Wright surveyed dozens of police chiefs, prison officials, and others to determine the extent of the drug problem in the United States. His 1909 survey focused on the problem of cocaine. Among six questions, the fourth dealt with the question of cocaine and crime: "What relation has the habitual use of the drug to crime?" The answers Wright received indicated a considerable lack of agreement. The police chief of Charleston, South Carolina, tersely replied that "in our experience" there was "not much" of a relationship.[34] The day before, however, the chief of police of Spokane, Washington, replied that "I never knew one to use it who was not a thief."[35]

What accounts for such divergence of opinion? It is possible, of course, that Charleston and Spokane had remarkably polar experiences with cocaine. The main source of disagreement was variable definitions of cocaine-related or cocaine-inspired crime. The Spokane chief, like many turn-of-the-century observers, had concluded that the crimes connected to cocaine users derived from their need to purchase the drug, crimes prompted especially by low economic status and exploitation of the consumer by drug retailers.[36] Scholars typically associate such criminal activity with the advent of prohibition and an illicit drug market. Yet prohibition of cocaine appears only to have accelerated a trend toward rising prices which began with the increase in popular consumption in the 1890s. Cocaine was never an inexpensive habit, and this proved especially problematic for the young and poor. The link between high cocaine prices and economic crime thus began as a preprohibition era phenomenon.

Dr. Alice Hamilton observed that the cocaine-using boys in the neighborhood of Hull House "would get so desperate for a dose that they would commit a crime to get it, hold up and rob, smash drugstore windows, intimidate drug clerks."[37] Catarrh cures introduced many young users to cocaine. When a druggist proved unwilling to sell pure cocaine, the catarrh cures might be the only available source of the drug. Catarrh cures were still a fairly expensive way to purchase cocaine, however, because users usually required several boxes of the product per week.[38] A cautionary tale in the *Medical Age* recounted the story of "a mere lad (aged fourteen) . . . advised to employ a certain proprietary remedy for catarrh," the young user began using two or three boxes of the cure per week. When he was forced to steal to obtain his supply, the editorial left no doubt what the inevitable products were: "Result: one ruined youth, a dishonored name, a heartbroken mother."[39]

Adult users, similarly unable to obtain their supply of cocaine, proved that stealing was hardly confined to young users of catarrh snuffs. The legal availability of cocaine was of small comfort to those without the means to purchase it. Even in the 1890s, before any formal regulation of distribution, cocaine sold for about 3¢ a grain at retail (often in packages costing 15¢ and containing 5 grains [325 milligrams] or packages costing 25¢ and containing 8 grains [520 milligrams]). Even under the best of circumstances, where retailers did not inflate their prices, dilute their product, or otherwise take advantage of their customers, a habitual user would have spent 30¢ a day to purchase 10 grains (650 milligrams) of cocaine.[40]

A habit that required even $2 per week, as with a 70-grain weekly habit, was in itself enough to strain the finances of many working-class, much less unemployed, users. But some of those identified as cocaine fiends used more than 10 grains per day. In 1896, Marks suggested that 12 to 15 grains (775–970 milligrams) per day was typical; Steinmetz claimed that addicts could use from 20 to 60 grains (1,300–3,900 milligrams) per day. Those addicted to morphine and cocaine in combination occasionally went on remarkable binges, consuming more than 100 grains (6,500 milligrams) in a single twenty-four-hour period![41]

Adding to the burden, cocaine addicts rarely found pure cocaine for only 3¢ a grain. The retail price of a "deck" (1.3 grains or about 85 milligrams) of cocaine in New York after 1908 was 25¢.[42] Inflated prices for cocaine were typical before 1908 as well. Users seeking to pay for costly habits sometimes became secondary distributors, adulterating their pure product to resell it at inflated prices. In many cities, adulterated cocaine (known on the street as *crown* in New Orleans and as *scrap* in Pittsburgh) became an important part of the supply.

Consequently, as one observer noted, "when a person has become an habitual user of cocaine he will steal anything that can be converted into money with which to purchase the drug." In 1914, pharmacists in Pittsburgh's East Liberty section were victimized by thieves who "under one pretext or another, succeeded in gaining access behind the prescription counter" to steal bottles of cocaine. In June of the same year, a downtown drugstore had a customer ask for cocaine. When he was refused, according to the *Western Pennsylvania Retail Druggist*, "the fellow became quite hysterical, and finally dropped upon his knees, and in a fervent prayer . . . asked that the good Lord would open the heart of the wicked drug clerk, and make him supply his need." Another druggist was threatened with a gun, and a woman "requested permission to go to the back of the prescription case to adjust her cloth-ing." The druggist "courteously remained in the front during the adjusting neces-sary, but afterwards discovered that his stock of cocaine had disappeared."[43]

When Hamilton Wright surveyed police chiefs in 1909 concerning the rela-tion of cocaine to crime, many referred only to crimes inspired by the need to pur-chase the drug. Sergeant Arthur Layne of the San Francisco Police Department told Wright that "after becoming addicted to its use, the victim will do anything, and commit any crime to get the drug, or the necessary money to purchase it." Layne also suggested that "when a person becomes a slave to the habit, he also becomes so incapacitated physically from earning a sufficient amount for the pur-chase of the drug and his own support, that he becomes a common thief." The view of the Wilkes-Barre, Pennsylvania, chief of police was that cocaine users were "addicted to committing larceny." Fred Kohler, then chief of police in Cleveland, told Wright that cocaine users were found among "all classes" but that "it [co-caine] causes many to steal in order to procure the drug."[44]

Harry Lewis, district attorney of Kings County, New York, addressed the sub-ject in a speech entitled "Is the Use of Habit-Forming Drugs a Crime Breeder?" Lewis divided drug-related crime into "those crimes which the addict commits in connection with the drug itself; that is, crimes having to do with its illicit traffic by dealers, and crimes committed by the addicts themselves," and criminal acts "which have nothing to do with the drug itself, but which are committed by the addict under circumstances which lead us to believe would not have been com-mitted if the drug had not been taken." "Eliminating the first," Lewis argued, "I find that very little remains. Most of the crimes committed as a result of taking drugs have been committed for the purpose of getting more drugs."

According to Lewis, every one of the drug-addicted inmates at Sing Sing state prison had been sent there after convictions for larcenies that had been commit-ted to provide "funds to buy more drugs." Directing his comments to those who argued that cocaine and other drugs had the effect of creating violent and crimi-nal behavior, he claimed to be unconvinced "that the use of the drug produces in the addict a desire to embrace the wrong in preference to the right, where the wrong be contrary to his individual nature." Rather, Lewis argued, "habitual use of narcotics merely weakens the will and possibly dulls the ability of the patient to distinguish the difference between right and wrong, but certainly makes him an easy prey to temptation and leads him to sometimes adopt criminal methods as the easiest way to make a living."[45]

Cocaine itself did not create the conditions described by Lewis and others. Rather, the high price of a cocaine habit combined with already marginal social and economic status to present very real dangers to some of the preprohibition users of the drug. Prominent among their concerns were the steady stream of entanglements with a variety of governmental institutions, including law enforcement, courts, and public health agencies, all of which increasingly defined cocaine use as a public issue. In the process, the relatively benign image of the medical-era "victim" of cocaine gave way to the pleasure-using cocaine fiend, whose vicious habits required a heightened level of supervision and control.

Images of the Cocaine Predator

Harry Lewis, while attacking the idea that the criminality of drug users could in any way be attributed to psychopharmacological effects, did allow for one exception to the rule: a young man named Dunn. "A hard working man without any previous criminal record" and employed in a restaurant, "without any apparent motive, went to a restaurant on Fulton Street, in Brooklyn . . . shot the restaurant keeper in cold blood, ran down the street, met a police officer, and without . . . hesitation turned and killed this officer." According to Lewis, the defendant testified that he had been using cocaine around the time of the murder. Physicians testified for the defense that Dunn's "ability to resist temptation had been destroyed" and that he could not have formed the necessary intent to make him guilty of the crime. According to Lewis, the "case is peculiar in my experience because the drug does seem to have been the direct cause of the crime."[46]

Lewis argued that Dunn's case was the exception to the rule and that cocaine users who committed crimes nearly always did so for the purposes of obtaining more cocaine. More importantly, Lewis and others did not believe that cocaine caused any fundamental change in the orientation of its users toward or away from violent crime. Not everyone shared this viewpoint. Edward Swann, district attorney for neighboring New York County, disagreed with Lewis, arguing that "the use of narcotic habit-forming drugs destroys the will power of the taker and when the will power of the individual is destroyed you leave the brute."[47] Whatever their actual number, the image of violent men like Dunn was central in the public perception of the dangers of cocaine; indeed, that Dunn himself offered his cocaine use in self-defense indicates the extent to which the violent effects of cocaine had become an accepted medicolegal concept in the turn-of-the-century discourse on drugs.

Explanations for the violent behavior of some cocaine users incorporated one or more of several related factors. First, some chronic cocaine users displayed what today might be called a kind of paranoid psychosis. This reaction, although not necessarily violent in itself, was thought to produce some violent encounters. Second, cocaine, as Alexander Lambert remarked, gave its users "a tremendous inflation of personality" and feelings of herculean strength and energy, which stimulated violent impulses. Third, cocaine caused a fundamental loss of control in the user, which could be manifested in countless ways, including violent behavior. Drug addiction specialist T. D. Crothers' explanation of the cocaine/violence connection illustrates the incorporation of these different perspectives into a larger theory of user behavior. Arguing that "criminality and lawless conduct" were "natural results" of cocaine use, Crothers pointed to the resulting "delusions of persecution" and the loss of "all ethical sense of law and order." In his view, the lower-class criminal who acted "wildly and maniacally" was probably "suffering from cocainism."[48]

More so than opiates, cocaine was said to lead its users into a variety of unpredictable and antisocial behaviors. In his well-known book, *The Individual Delinquent,* William Healy argued for a substantial relationship between cocaine use and criminality. Although he acknowledged that cocaine use among juveniles was relatively infrequent, he offered one case to demonstrate the destructive impact of cocaine on health and morals, a case worth citing in full:

> Case 29, was reported to us as being certainly that of a cocainist. This was a boy of distinctly inferior type, coming from a notoriously bad environment, who had cocaine in his possession. He was an excessive thief and vagrant, associating with the lowest companions. He glibly gave an account of the most miserable forms of life in the underworld. Already at 15 he had had two venereal diseases. Offered a helping hand by a manly police officer, he was so weak willed that he could not lift himself out of the mire, although he steadily maintained that he wished to do better. His word was absolutely unreliable. In court this boy took on the toughest attitudes, and volubly insisted that he was being persecuted by the police. He had been already 4 times in the adult courts through always giving his wrong age, and, although small in size, had twice served terms in adult houses of correction.
>
> Chiefly notable about him was his poor physical condition, his lack of will power, his excessive lying, and his attitude of boldness.
>
> It is well recognized that some criminals, and rarely others, take this drug to give them physical steadiness and temporarily heighten their mental capacity. Occasionally a criminal will become so far influenced by it that he loses all foresight and self-control, and is ready to shoot to kill upon the slightest provocation. If we saw the case cited above a few years later we should probably find him a most dangerous fellow, carrying weapons, and willing to do anything desperate.[49]

This particular example illustrates the murky connections between cocaine and other deviant behaviors. Healy suggested that the case demonstrated the impact of cocaine addiction, but the evidence he presented revealed nothing more than possession of cocaine. Even had Case 29 been a cocaine addict, it is difficult to say what aspects of his lifestyle and behavior (thievery, vagrancy, bad associations, venereal disease, "attitude of boldness," lying) Healy felt were a direct result of the drug.[50]

The connection between cocaine and violence presents a complicated historical problem, where perception and reality are difficult to disentangle. Real incidents of violent and erratic behavior associated with nonmedical cocaine use almost surely did occur, much as they did in various doctors' offices during the medical era. Indeed, in a summary of seventeen cases of cocaine addiction published in 1893, J. B. Mattison described a wide range of behavioral changes. One young professional "could scarcely restrain himself from assaulting imaginary tormentors, with whom he remonstrated on the street"; another addict assaulted patients at the hospital where he was being treated; and a physician "became violent and vowed to kill himself or others who might try to restrain him."[51] Yet the image of the violent cocaine-crazed menace seems to have been just that: an image, fed by a few violent episodes and sustained by fear and prejudice. As the idea of the cocaine fiend spread, it may have provided a construct by which real violence could be made intelligible.

Nowhere was this more true than in the South, where police departments in particular rallied to the defense of white communities against supposed cocaine-crazed blacks. No one expressed a more extreme view than Edward Huntington Williams, whose efforts to scare his northern readers away from alcohol prohibition have already been noted. Cocaine, Williams believed, transformed "hitherto inoffensive, law abiding negroes" into "a constant menace to his community." Under the influence of cocaine, "sexual desires are increased and perverted, peaceful negroes become quarrelsome, and timid negroes develop a degree of 'Dutch courage' that is sometimes almost incredible." The result was that "a large proportion of the wholesale killings in the South during recent years have been the result of cocaine." A black user of cocaine was "absolutely beyond redemption."[52]

Not only did cocaine destroy the moral sense of the black user, according to Williams, but the drug endowed its users with a nearly superhuman strength. Southern law enforcement officers increased the caliber of their guns in light of the idea that, as Williams described it, "the cocaine nigger is sure hard to kill." In support of this thesis, Williams offered little more than a chilling story from D. K. Lyerly, police chief of Asheville, North Carolina. Fighting with a black man he attempted to arrest, Lyerly drew his gun and fired, "for I knew I had to kill him quick." As Williams described it, "this bullet did not even stagger the crazed negro, and neither did a second bullet which pierced the biceps muscle and entered the thorax," so the officer finally had to "finish the man with his club." The following day Mr. Lyerly exchanged his .32–20 for a .38 caliber army model. Williams followed this graphic passage with other examples designed to show that "cocaine, besides making the habitué homicidal, adds to his ability to carry out the homicidal intent" by improving, rather than impairing, his marksmanship.[53]

Williams stated that "ever since the emancipation of the slaves the South has been confronted by a problem that does not exist in the North. This problem is the control of the negro — particularly the low-class negro." In such an overheated environment, mythical black crime waves flourished. Not long after the peak of an epidemic of lynching, amid fears of black rapists, a drug that reputedly broke down self-control could be readily attacked, and isolated violent incidents could quickly become legendary. A crime story in one county was often quickly reprinted in graphic detail in newspapers throughout the region.[54]

Two separate incidents exemplify the legend of cocaine-inspired violence in the making. The first incident took place in New Orleans and involved a nationally publicized shooting spree and a subsequent race riot in July 1900. As noted previously, New Orleans in 1900 had already seen cocaine use become quite prevalent. In that climate, Robert Charles, a black man, could easily be accused of being a cocaine fiend after he went on a shooting spree that left seven people (including three police officers) dead and twenty others wounded. The reasons for Charles' attacks remain rather vague, but white New Orleans was ready to provide its own explanations. There is no actual proof that Charles was under the influence of cocaine, yet various newspapers claimed that police found a "bottle of cocaine" or a "box" of cocaine in his residence.[55] In this instance, otherwise incomprehensible behavior could be explained comfortably by the supposed degenerative effects of the drug.

The second incident occurred in Mississippi in the small Yazoo Valley town of Harriston, not far from Natchez. Like New Orleans, this region of Mississippi had witnessed the recent proliferation of cocaine. In September 1913, two brothers, Walter and Will Jones, were accused of having shot and killed three persons, including a former constable and the sheriff of Jefferson County. That the victims were white and the shooters black caused a furious uproar, during which Will was lynched, and his brother was shot. An ensuing race riot was suppressed only by the arrival of a company of National Guardsmen from Natchez. The dead brothers were immediately accused of having been under the influence of cocaine; the prominence that this feature of the story was given may be observed in the headline of the *New York Herald:* "10 Killed, 35 Hurt in Race Riot

Born of a Cocaine 'Jag.' "[56] The Mississippi violence came as Congress considered an early version of the Harrison Narcotic Act. Defending his support of the measure to a physician back home, South Carolina Senator Ben Tillman, a veteran of racial politics, pointed to the problems cocaine was said to cause among blacks. "I suppose you saw in the papers some days ago," Tillman wrote, "where the two mulatto boys in Harriston, Mississippi, got crazed on cocaine and went on the war path with the result that eight people were killed and a large number wounded."[57]

Public opinion about the link between cocaine and violence was shaped by the widespread publicity given to notorious cases. The stories were shocking, but few questioned whether they were representative (or accurate). In another widely quoted example, a Louisville physician cited a white male cocaine addict who "while walking over a high viaduct . . . met a little girl and her baby brother, and without any warning he seized the little girl and hurled her over the railing to the rocks about seventy feet below." Like the example of the murderous Dunn, this man also employed in his self-defense his use of cocaine.[58] In New Orleans, the district attorney reported the case of Edward Ramey (also white), who beat a jeweler to death while under the influence of cocaine. Whether or not cocaine had anything to do with either of these two notorious crimes, the publicity surrounding them did much to reinforce the public understanding of cocaine users as predictably violent.[59]

In exploring the historical link between cocaine and crime, drug-induced violent behavior accounted for relatively few of the crimes for which cocaine users were held responsible. Most users in the urban underground ran afoul of the law fairly regularly but almost entirely for various minor offenses. No doubt, as was widely charged, the high cost of legally available cocaine compelled some users to resort to theft or burglary to obtain it. Violent cocaine fiends, however, appear to have been more a terrifying social fiction than an empirical reality and one with a sharp racial overtone. Especially in the racially tense South, but also in the cities of the North, such fears flourished and shaped the prevalent image of the cocaine user as an unpredictable menace to social order.

Clearly, the image of turn-of-the-century drug users as secure in their right to privacy, relatively content and unmolested, does not square with the more complex historical reality. An overreliance by historians on legislative milestones, especially the start of legal prohibition, is at least partly responsible for oversimplifying the record. The extent to which local authorities dealt with cocaine abusers and "coke drunks" reflects an important aspect of state involvement in the lives of cocaine users which historians have largely overlooked. Although most states failed to pass any kind of legislation regulating users until the end of the first decade of the twentieth century, new legislation mainly confirmed patterns of enforcement begun earlier, especially via aggressive use of vagrancy laws. That governmental efforts were unsystematic and certainly unsympathetic in no way diminishes their importance as indicators of active state involvement in the preprohibition era.

SEVEN

The Cautionary Tale
Cocaine and Drug Industry Regulation

Shortly before Christmas 1909, federal food and drug inspector J. L. Lynch arrived in New Orleans to conduct an investigation. For most of that year Lynch had been assisting the Bureau of Chemistry in its prosecution of various soft drink manufacturers, most notably Coca-Cola, for violations of the Pure Food and Drug Act of 1906. Lynch met with several of the physicians who had testified in the first Coca-Cola trial, and all repeated their strong condemnations of the drink. One of the doctors informed Lynch that several clothing manufacturers in the city were in the habit of keeping their young female employees "supplied in Coca-Cola." Armed with this information, Lynch visited two overall manufacturers. At the second, the superintendent told Lynch that the firm, which employed four hundred people, had allowed one young man to have Coca-Cola delivered to the factory, where he would distribute the drinks and keep the profit. Under this arrangement, three to five cases of two dozen bottles were sold each day, with some employees consuming four to six bottles a day.

Under further questioning by Lynch, the superintendent acknowledged that the firm had discontinued the practice six months earlier. Selling the Coca-Cola had become somewhat of a distraction, and one of the owners had concluded that the drink "was a detriment to the help." At present, then, the women were not permitted to purchase the beverage during regular working hours, but when overtime was required, nearly all of them asked for permission to go out and get a "dope" before returning to work. The superintendent concluded his conversation with Lynch by observing "that this drink was a habit-forming one, as he had noticed that it was almost always the same crowd of his help who drank it." Lynch then relayed all of this information to Dr. W. G. Campbell, chief inspector for the Bureau of Chemistry.[1]

In his travels through New Orleans, Lynch encountered a citizenry for whom the language of drugs and drug using had become almost commonplace. The shopgirls who asked for a "dope" when they purchased Coca-Cola, the doctors who advised their patients against consuming the soft drink, and the superintendent who identified a Coca-Cola habit among his workers posed a hard question: was there a relationship between the emergence of the menacing cocaine fiend and the popular sale and use of many products in which coca or cocaine was an ingredient?

In answering this question in the affirmative, Lynch joined a growing anticocaine coalition intent upon restricting public access to the drug. The drive for cocaine control became an important part of a wider Progressive Era movement to regulate the development and distribution of new drug products (Figure 7.1). In the hard-fought campaign to create a regulatory apparatus for the drug industry, the American cocaine experience served reformers well as an object lesson — a cautionary tale — about the dangers inherent in an unregulated drug industry.

From the start, the close relationship of the anticocaine and drug-regulation activists meant that early control measures would reflect dual motives. One motive centered on minimizing the harms generated by widespread availability. Reformers whose central focus was the reduction of cocaine abuse encompassed the fields of public health, child welfare, social work, and temperance — a list that only begins to suggest the diversity of the reform movement. The second motive was the creation of a basic system of drug regulation. For would-be drug regulators, cocaine was but one example — albeit a very powerful one — of the need to bring a legal order to the pharmaceutical industry. The American Medical Association (AMA), the most influential of the advocates for reform, claimed that the cocaine experience demonstrated that commercial interests, left uncontrolled, would always win out over "medical science" and public safety. Both groups were joined by an unlikely ally — the leading ethical drug manufacturers, willing to abandon their interest in cocaine and coca products in order to influence new legislation in a direction that favored them over the patent medicine industry.

Working together, this coalition produced a series of controls over the capacity of the pharmaceutical industry to deliver cocaine to the consumer. The results of its efforts appear to have been as mixed as its motives. Reformers were able to eliminate from the market most packaged medicines and tonics containing cocaine and to do so even before passage of the federal Harrison Narcotic Act in 1914 launched national drug prohibition. More importantly, using cocaine as powerful example of industry indifference to public health, the AMA, leading ethical drug manufacturers, and the federal government asserted substantive new powers over drug development and distribution.

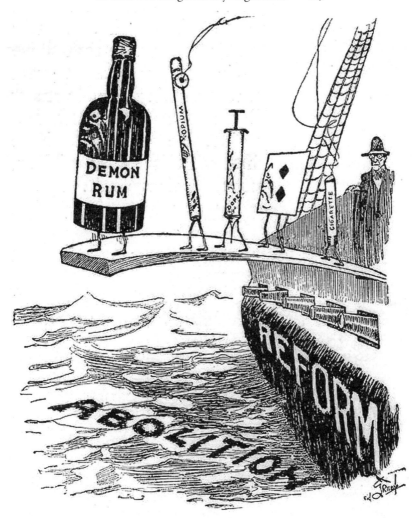

Figure 7.1. Progressive Era temperance. Although the cocaine control movement had distinct characteristics, many observers saw a direct connection to Progressive Era temperance movements generally. Here, "dope" walks the plank of abolition with cigarettes, a playing card, an opium pipe, and demon rum. *New York Telegram.*

A Coalition for Control Emerges

The Pure Food and Drug Act of 1906, which provided the authority for Lynch's New Orleans investigation, was merely one legislative product of a much larger effort aimed at regulating the manufacture of drugs and medical products. Indeed, the strength of the control coalition did not fully manifest itself in the resulting legislation, under which state regulatory and police powers remained notoriously weak. The true measure of its influence was the capacity to shape public opinion and to control the flow of information regarding the drug industry and product safety. To achieve these ambitious ends, three groups, each of which considered cocaine a useful example of why regulation was required, came together in powerful coalition.

The first group consisted of muckraking journalists, whose sensational articles claimed to expose the nefarious and dangerous practices of patent medicine makers. With their secret compositions and disdain for organized medicine, these manufacturers seemed the very embodiment of the sinister corporate interests that sought profit at the expense of American public health. By far the best known of these writers was Samuel Hopkins Adams, whose series in *Collier's* is considered a classic example of the muckraking genre. *The Great American Fraud,* as Adams styled it, included the sale of "cocain- and opium-bearing nostrums." Accepting the negative imagery of the drug fiend, Adams and other writers condemned a trade that "makes criminals of our young men and harlots of our young women."[2]

The second locus of reform activity was the federal government, especially the Department of Agriculture and its Bureau of Chemistry, headed by Harvey W. Wiley. It was Wiley who helped fight for passage of the Pure Food and Drug Act in 1906, and it was Wiley who subsequently administered it. He had been head of the Department of Agriculture Division of Chemistry since 1883 and had spent years urging Congress to pass legislation to curb what he regarded as the underhanded practices of food and drug manufacturers.

The earliest and ultimately most powerful voices for control were reform-minded physicians and their professional organizations, most notably the AMA. Relatively weak and ineffectual in the nineteenth century, the AMA claimed greater authority over the medical profession by the start of the twentieth century. In 1905, the AMA organized the Council on Pharmacy and Chemistry, a regulatory group intended to raise consciousness about dangerous or ineffective remedies.

Physicians, particularly those charged with responsibility for safeguarding professional identity and authority, recognized that they had been unable to establish an acceptable level of control over the distribution and use of new drug products. Nathan S. Davis of the AMA was an important advocate of the Pure Food and Drug Act of 1906 and was among those responsible for establishing the AMA Council on Pharmacy and Chemistry. The purpose of the council was to provide an official stamp of approval for all drug products; a company risked disapproval if it made specific therapeutic claims, failed to disclose ingredients, or advertised directly to the public. In that same year, Davis argued that physicians "cannot blame manufacturing chemists for finding new things or advertising them as cleverly as possible." "That they and the nostrum vendor are surprisingly successful in selling their wares," Davis concluded, "is largely our fault."[3] Davis suggested that physicians had allowed drug manufacturers and retailers to control information regarding drug efficacy and use. Through this control, drug manufacturers had been able to achieve a measure of public trust and legitimacy which Davis and other physicians clearly felt they did not deserve.

Physicians made similar observations about the control of cocaine in particular. Lewis Mason, physician and president of the American Association for the Study of Inebriety, observed in 1902 that it was partly the failure of the medical profession to control the distribution of new products which was responsible for the spread of cocaine abuse: "too often the child of the laboratory is a product not only for good but frequently for evil, so that we might almost say, 'Would that it had never been born.'"[4]

Mason's solution in 1902 was to challenge the ability of manufacturers to sell products that physicians determined were dangerous. Anticipating legislation to come, Mason proposed a three-part approach. First, the individual states or the federal government should appoint a chemist to analyze all drug preparations and determine their contents. Second, the state could refuse to issue a patent or proprietary right for any products found to contain "dangerous" drugs. Finally, Mason urged "heavy penalties of fine or imprisonment" if such products were sold, the penalties applying to both manufacturer and retailer.[5]

To a great extent, the activities of reform groups overlapped, and each frequently found occasion to work with the other toward common regulatory and reform goals. The AMA, for example, reprinted and distributed more than one hundred thousand copies of Samuel Hopkins Adams' series. The AMA Bureau of Pharmacy and Chemistry, whose approval was necessary if a manufacturer wished to advertise a product in professional medical journals, counted as members Harvey Wiley and Lyman F. Kebler (chief of the Bureau of Chemistry drug division). Wiley himself was something of a muckraker, authoring a regular series in *Cosmopolitan* and working closely with various private reform organizations, including the Women's Christian Temperance Union.

Such a close relationship between public and private organizations in seeking to regulate cocaine distribution does not, however, indicate any grand or exceptional conspiracy to deprive consumers of cocaine. Rather, such a coalition typified Progressive Era reform mechanisms, in which superficially weak state authority was bolstered through public/private cooperation. If private organizations such as the AMA, for instance, worked to affect public legislation to their own advantage, they did so no more than countless other interest groups.

The Celery-Cola Case:
The Paradox of Cocaine Control

Friday afternoon, March 11, 1910, attorney John L. Stone spent six long hours in a Birmingham, Alabama, courtroom waiting for the jury to return a verdict for or against his clients, the makers of Celery-Cola. Five months earlier, agents of the Bureau of Chemistry had seized a shipment of the soft drink on its way to New Orleans. The bureau had Celery-Cola ("delicious," "refreshing," "pure," and "sold round the world" according to company advertising) analyzed and found that one glass of the beverage contained 0.002 grain of cocaine (about 0.03 milligram) and between 1.25 and 2 grains of caffeine (about 80–130 milligrams). Company president J. F. Hawkins, secretary and treasurer J. W. Altman, and stockholder J. G. Bradley were all charged with violations of the Pure Food and Drug Act of 1906; their trial revealed the mixed motives and ambiguous results of the anticocaine effort.[6]

The act under which the government prosecuted the Celery-Cola defendants required national labeling of all drug products and packaged medicines which would state the presence of cocaine in their products. In fact, section 8 of the act enumerated which drugs were specifically required to be identified: morphine, opium, cocaine, heroin, alpha or beta eucaine, chloroform, cannabis indica, chloral hydrate, or acetanilide, or any "derivative or preparation of any such substances." Although the act (administered by Harvey W. Wiley's Bureau of Chemistry) held out the possibility of dealing with false or misleading claims, initial enforcement focused largely on mislabeling. Section 7 of the Food and Drug Act also allowed claims of adulteration of food products, if the food "contained added ingredients which may render such product injurious to health"; cocaine was one such ingredient.

The prosecution of the Celery-Cola case had been preceded by, and took place in the context of, a vigorous and active publicity campaign against the use of cocaine in manufacture. Led by Harvey Wiley and the AMA, reformers showed little interest in presenting a restrained view of the cocaine problem in the United States. Dr. Lyman F. Kebler, chief of the Bureau of Chemistry drug division and member of the AMA Council on Pharmacy and Chemistry, had that same year made the preposterous estimate that "there were at present 6,000,000 cocaine victims in the United States." As if this figure did not seem troubling enough, Kebler noted that "in New York, where the 'dope fiend' is more numerous than in any other spot on earth, the police claim that certain sections of the city are literally rotten with the white poison and that fifty percent of the pickpockets, burglars, and thugs who infest the city and crowd the jails, are recruited from the cocaine dens." As Kebler wrote, the language of the "cocaine fiend" phenomenon merged with Progressive Era drug legislation.[7]

The coalition for control directed most of its considerable verbal fire at patent medicine makers, with little attention to distinguishing among companies or products. In the case of cocaine, its mere presence in a product was enough to demonstrate willful disregard for public health. Curiously, reformers seemed to save some of their harshest criticism for low-potency products such as Celery-Cola. Although Samuel Hopkins Adams acknowledged that catarrh cures were widely sold, misleadingly advertised, and frequently abused, he also took the time to single out Vin Mariani. Mariani's product, according to Adams, was a dangerous cocaine preparation. As he wrote in *Collier's* in 1907:

> In the sudden light which the Pure Food law throws into certain dark corners, that widely bruited pick-me-up for lassitudinous ladies, Vin Mariani, takes on a changed aspect. From the enthusiastic encomiums, given out for advertising purposes by sundry actresses, one might suppose that the so-called French preparation was at once the most bracing and the most harmless of concoctions. Across its label, however, the pure food law has recorded the warning fact: "Each ounce represents one-tenth of one grain of cocain."[8]

Lyman Kebler recalled Vin Mariani as a "very poisonous product."[9] The AMA was even harder on Mariani; a subcommittee of the Council on Pharmacy and Chemistry concluded that the company was guilty of "gross misrepresentations and fraud" and of making untrue therapeutic claims for its wine. The AMA even questioned the veracity of the endorsements that Mariani distributed, including that of former President William McKinley ("think of it!" exclaimed the author of the report), suggesting that they might be "fakes."[10]

Through its enforcement of the Pure Food and Drug Act, the Bureau of Chemistry evinced considerable hostility for relatively harmless, low-potency products. Ignoring the pleas of manufacturers that coca leaves contained variable amounts of cocaine, the bureau insisted that coca products indicate the precise cocaine content on their labels, making the use of coca and fluid extract of coca exceedingly difficult. Even more significant was Wiley's decision to utilize the food adulteration provisions of section 7 to great effect against soft drinks, simply by classifying the beverages as food products. Although the makers of soft drinks such as Koca-Nola *did* violate the law by claiming to be "dopeless" and by failing to note the presence of cocaine in their product, it was also true that Koca-Nola contained less than 1 milligram of cocaine per full glass. Indeed, of all of the patent medicines the federal government ever pursued, none was attacked more aggressively than the Coca-Cola Company, with which the government engaged in years of litigation.[11]

An attorney for the Coca-Cola Company, upon hearing that the Celery-Cola case was under way, hurried to Birmingham from Atlanta. Arriving on the second and last day of the trial, the attorney helped John L. Stone craft his closing arguments to the jury.[12] Testimony on the first day included the government chemist H. C. Fuller (formerly employed by both Parke, Davis and Mallinckrodt), who testified to the presence of cocaine and caffeine. The government then brought forward a series of doctors willing to testify to the harmfulness of both drugs to the human body. The examination of the doctors by U.S. Attorney O. D. Street brought forth a curious mix of pharmacology and folklore, intended to damn Celery-Cola as a threat to the general welfare. Questioning of Dr. W. B. Parks produced the following exchange:

Q. If long continued, even in small doses, what effect will it [cocaine] have upon the nervous system?

A. It has a very bad nervous depressing effect upon the general system. If continued it will make the patient very anemic and nervous, and if continued very long the patient is apt to have hallucinations. It causes destruction of the brain cells, and that produces insanity.

Q. And what effect does it have upon the moral faculties of the victim? (Objection by counsel for defendants, on ground that question is immaterial, irrelevant, and incompetent. Objection overruled. Exception noted.)

A. It has a very bad effect on the moral faculties, very quickly.

Q. Now doctor, you say that the effect of that habit is to break down the moral faculties of the victim, I will ask you if that effect is to excite lustful desires? (Objection by counsel for defendants, on ground that question is immaterial, irrelevant, and incompetent. Objection overruled.)

A. In some it does and some it does not. In some it increases desire and in some it entirely obliterates it.

Q. Have you observed among which race of people it is that this cocaine habit is most prevalent?

(Objection by counsel for defendants, on ground that question is immaterial, irrelevant, and incompetent. Objection overruled. Exception noted.)

A. Well, it is prevalent in both races, but it seems that the negro takes to it very readily.[13]

The next day, after deliberating for six hours, the jury returned a verdict of guilty, and the judge imposed a $25 fine on the defendants.

The trial of the Celery-Cola makers must certainly have been about more than simply the enforcement of restrictive legislation. A $25 fine would scarcely have been sufficient to deter would-be violators, and the small quantities of cocaine could hardly have been the danger prosecution witnesses claimed. Moreover, by the time of the trial, the Celery-Cola Company had already voluntarily replaced the fluid extract coca in its Celery-Cola formula with tea and argued to the Bureau of Chemistry that "the publication of the assay you give of Celery-Cola can result in nothing but injustice to us." Publicizing the small amount of cocaine, the company argued, "can have no corrective effect for correction has already been made; it will be misleading and cause us much harm, both financial and personal; it will be deceiving to the public, which is the very thing your department is fighting against."[14] Nevertheless, the assay of Celery-Cola was published by the government and reprinted and widely distributed by the AMA.

As the government's own summary of the case stated, the intent was to demonstrate that cocaine "was a drug which should never be administered in . . . a product which was available for all persons at all times."[15] By this standard, no exceptions were possible. To enforce this standard, public opinion needed to be aroused. In one sure sign of its success, soft drinks became closely associated in public discourse with the cocaine habit. W. A. Starnes, proprietor of a drug treatment sanitarium in Atlanta, believed that "cocoa cola is doing more injury to the human race than all other drugs put together."[16] A 1912 film directed by D. W. Griffith featured a father and son whose lives were disrupted by the cocaine soft drink business the father had started.[17] J. Leyden White's pamphlet, "The Coca-Cola 'Joker' in the Harrison Narcotic Law," offered the public a rambling diatribe against the Coca-Cola Company for including cocaine in its product. White accused the company of creating Coca-Cola addicts at the soda fountain.[18] Soft drink manufacturers indirectly acknowledged the problem in their advertising; Wiseola, for example, proclaimed itself "free from qualities that would tend to create habit."[19] Other companies exploited the controversy; the Dr. Pepper Company of Waco, Texas, not only advertised its products as "free from caffein and other drugs," the firm's president collected information on Coca-Cola habitués and offered the material to J. L. Lynch when his investigation moved from New Orleans to Texas.[20]

The Drug Industry Concedes the Cocaine Issue

As the control coalition's challenge to the drug industry intensified, the notable feature of the industry response was its willingness to abandon the use of cocaine. Just as reformers recognized that the popularity of the drug as an ingredient in tonics and medicines could be used to establish the need for regulation, many drug makers easily discarded the drug. Indeed, by the time the Harrison Narcotic Act went into effect in 1915, nearly all of the coca and cocaine products were gone. The dozens of wines, soft drinks, tonics, and snuffs vanished from the shelves of American drugstores nearly as fast as they had first appeared. Those products that survived, such as Vin Mariani and Coca-Cola, did so in new, "decocainized" versions.

What killed this vast array of products? For the most part, the willingness of manufacturers to concede the cocaine issue to the social reformers ensured the end of the cocaine product lines. Motivations, of course, differed from company to company. For some business owners, perhaps, the condemnations of cocaine struck a responsive chord. For others, the fear of prosecution and negative publicity surely offered motivation enough to de-cocainize their business. In most cases, however, the financial significance of cocaine simply failed to keep pace with the changing climate of the modern drug industry, where new synthetic drugs emerged rapidly as the primary source of profit. Particularly in the case of the ethical drug business, straining to demonstrate its scientific integrity, cocaine was worth more dead than alive.

Ethical firms might accept inevitable regulation, hoping to influence its content, but most industry figures never really saw the need for government supervision. Albert B. Lyons, the first chemist Parke, Davis had employed, looked back in 1926 on forty years of industry experience and concluded that "90 percent of legal enactments have in them the character of injustice which ought to prevent their adoption, and frequently condemns them in the court as unconstitutional."[21] H. K. Mulford, whose firm competed with Parke, Davis through World War I for the title of *leading* scientific pharmaceutical manufacturer, felt that a reliance on corporate integrity was the central question: "a physician is no more interested in knowing how a pharmaceutical or chemical is made . . . than he is in knowing where the iron comes from that goes into his steel instruments." For Mulford the matter was ultimately one of trust. After the creation of the Council on Pharmacy and Chemistry, Mulford complained that "the trouble with these self-constituted bodies . . . is the fact that they do not give credit to the manufacturer of having any basic moral principle."[22]

Ironically, the growing capacity of the ethical industry for research and development of new drug products actually sped the decline of cocaine's place in the business through the discovery and aggressive marketing of various synthetic alternatives. Firms such as Smith, Kline & French in Philadelphia, Sharpe & Dohme in Baltimore, and Eli Lilly & Company in Indianapolis, which had operated for years as dealers and distributors of plant-based pharmaceutical products, emerged as dealers in new alkaloid and synthetic drugs with nationwide markets. At the same time, these firms began channeling profits into research divisions to develop new products. Newer firms emerged, such as the H. K. Mulford Company, with a primary commitment to scientific research in the pursuit of profitable new drugs.[23]

For these rapidly developing ethical enterprises, cocaine lost much of the luster it had in the late nineteenth century. Much of the problem stemmed from growing medical conservatism in the use of cocaine, which restricted the opportunity for marketing the drug in medical circles. Moreover, after the initial flurry of new medical applications for cocaine which followed Koller's work, few new uses for the drug had been developed. This was not for lack of effort on the part of some firms, most notably Parke, Davis. In a company publication from the mid 1890s, Parke, Davis editorially acknowledged the task at hand: "the pharmacology of cocaine has received much attention and is pretty well worked out. But it still remains for us to make it a valuable and serviceable remedy."[24]

Older patterns of product development clearly failed to win much acceptance within the industry. Returning from one of his subsequent trips to coca-growing regions, botanist Henry Hurd Rusby brought home to Parke, Davis a coca elixir that he had found to be "in great vogue" as an after-dinner liqueur in La Paz. Impressed with the ability of the elixir to aid in digestion, Rusby believed he had found a potentially popular preparation. Finding interest at the company somewhat muted, Rusby approached the British firm of Burroughs & Wellcome, and although they expressed some initial interest, he found they "began to appreciate the dangers in the use of this drug, and the idea was never carried out."[25]

With the development of a more recognizably modern research capacity, firms such as Parke, Davis sought new medical products in which cocaine might be employed usefully; the results were dismal. Often these efforts involved cocaine in combination with other drugs. The company attempted to design a new anesthetic by using cocaine in combination with a new product called Chloretone. The new preparation did very poorly; in fact, the company declared the new combination a "disaster."[26] In 1899, the company developed a hypodermic tablet with cocaine, strychnine, and nitroglycerin.[27] Around 1904, the firm began experimental work with compounds of cocaine and adrenaline. Parke, Davis had only recently been responsible for the introduction of adrenaline, and the company recognized that its popular new drug might be combined with cocaine. In 1906 their research resulted in the production of an adrenaline and cocaine hypodermic tablet.[28] The H. K. Mulford Company, main rival to Parke, Davis in the field of scientific research, called its version Adrin-Cocaine. Neither effort was a success, and Parke, Davis dropped its product, the last of the new cocaine ventures, in 1918.

Pharmaceutical research did far better in finding synthetic substitutes for cocaine than in finding new uses for it. In April 1896, the European pharmaceutical firm Schering & Glatz introduced a synthetic replacement, eucaine, to the United States. Schering's product proved immediately popular with physicians as an effective anesthetic. Unlike earlier efforts at producing synthetic substitutes, Schering could offer its product at $3.50 an ounce, the same cost as cocaine.[29] Even more damaging to the use of cocaine by physicians was the marketing of procaine (Novocain) by Farbwerke Hoescht. Hoescht, through its American marketing agents, advertised its product by making explicit comparisons with cocaine. In a 1907 advertisement in the *Oil, Paint, and Drug Reporter,* the company described the advantages of its product:

> NOVOCAIN. A Definite Chemical, Not a Mixture. Perfect Substitute for Cocain. Relatively Nontoxic, Nonirritating. Anesthesia as profound and more prolonged. Ten times less toxic than Cocain. DOES NOT PRODUCE HABIT.

Hoescht also traded on the support for alternatives to cocaine among the medical profession, noting that Novocain had been "approved by the Council on Chemistry and Pharmacy AMA."[30] Products such as Novocain reduced the use of cocaine as an anesthetic, the main area in which physicians still valued cocaine after the turn of the century. Despite the efforts of the leading pharmaceutical research laboratories, no effective or salable cocaine compounds emerged to reinvigorate interest in the drug among physicians.

As new experimentation waned, firms such as Parke, Davis gradually trimmed their existing lines of products, especially the coca preparations that had formerly been so popular but now seemed out of step with modern pharmaceutical science. In 1905, the company replaced the kola and coca in its Celery-Cola compound with equivalent amounts of caffeine and cocaine. Soon afterward, the company dropped many coca items, including the powdered and solid extracts of coca, and the Coca, Beef, and Iron Wine (in 1907).[31] Interest in such products was dampened further by state requirements that cocaine and coca products be labeled as poisons. Thus, boxes of Birney's Catarrh Cure sold in New York bore labels reading: "This preparation, containing among other valuable ingredients, a small quantity of COCAINE, is, in accordance with the New York Pharmacy act, hereby labeled POISON!"[32] As with the Pure Food and Drug Act, few state poison regulations made any distinction among various amounts of cocaine in products. Consequently, many products with little appeal to cocaine habitués fell under the labeling provisions. O. W. Smith, head of the Parke, Davis New York operations, worried that applying red and white poison labels to the company's voice tablets, in compliance with New York and New Jersey laws, "would practically render them unsalable."[33]

Even more than the ethical firms, the patent medicine makers strongly resisted the imposition of government regulation. Yet here, too, most companies found it expedient to end their use of coca and cocaine. It had become readily apparent to the industry that neither the government nor the reform press made much distinction among various types of product in which cocaine was an ingredient. Harvey Wiley made the point quite directly to one manufacturer's attorney, advising that "we don't care about the amount [of cocaine in the product] — the amount makes absolutely no difference."[34] This, drug makers knew, was technically true: because the Pure Food and Drug Act was authorized only to judge whether a product was misbranded or adulterated, the quantity of cocaine made little difference. In this climate, tonics, coca wines, voice tablets, and the William A. Webster Company antivomiting tablets found themselves exposed to the same penalties as the potent catarrh cures.

The public image problem this situation presented for the manufacturers was considerable. Most had extensive lines of medical products which they did not want compromised by negative publicity over a single product. The experience of the Maltine Company typifies the response of the patent medicine business. Established in the mid nineteenth century in Brooklyn, the company's leading products were the popular tonic beverage Maltine and many combinations of Maltine with other ingredients. When the benefits of coca and then cocaine were publicized in the 1880s, Maltine added "Maltine with Coca." By the early twentieth century, the Maltine Company was emerging as a patent medicine manufacturer with serious ambitions to be accepted by the medical profession as an ethical firm. As early as 1894, the firm had responded to complaints from physicians about its advertising by arguing, in a letter to various medical journals, that "Maltine is distinctly not a 'patent medicine,' nor has it ever been advertised to the public . . . we have statistics to prove that 90 percent of the physicians of the United

States prescribe Maltine . . . we reach the patient *only through the physician.*[35] Eventually the Maltine Company became Chilcott Laboratories, now part of the Warner Lambert Company.[36]

Maltine Coca Wine was fairly popular, with more than ten thousand bottles sold annually; yet the product was withdrawn in September 1907 in response to growing public scrutiny of patent medicines containing cocaine. Each bottle contained perhaps a few milligrams of cocaine, although the precise amounts were too small to be measured accurately. Nevertheless, as the Maltine attorney explained to the Bureau of Chemistry, the product was withdrawn "simply because all these cocaine preparations are getting into such bad odor that the Maltine Company doesn't want anything to do with one . . . we thought it advisable to be on the safe side and give up the preparation altogether rather than get mixed up in anything unpleasant." One bureau member, noting that Maltine with Coca had only trace amounts of cocaine, inquired, "why should you care about any attitude against cocaine preparations? You say your chemists have not been able to detect any cocaine." The Maltine attorney could only respond that "anything with the label 'Coca Wine' is objected to by most people . . . we feel it would hurt our other products to have a coca wine on the market."[37]

Other companies responded similarly by eliminating cocaine from the product rather than eliminating the product altogether. Coca-Cola and most of its soft drink–producing counterparts voluntarily eliminated the trace amounts of cocaine in their products by switching to de-cocainized coca leaves — the residue coca from the cocaine manufacturing process, purchased from chemical companies. The Wiseola Company assured the government that "until 1909, we used the extract of Coca leaves, which had not gone through this process, and the Chemist has not been able to find any trace of cocain, so we feel sure that our product at this time contains no trace of cocain."[38]

Patent medicine makers were also somewhat dependent on the willingness of ethical companies to aid in the manufacture of coca and cocaine products. Ethical firms such as Parke, Davis had long maintained profitable business manufacturing patent medicines for other companies such as Dr. Elder's Tobacco Specific, a tobacco-habit cure that contained some cocaine. The intense pressure on cocaine, however, led to a reconsideration of this enterprise. In a stern letter written in 1910, Parke, Davis warned one Southern soft drink manufacturer against ordering fluid extract of coca from them: "we manufacture and sell FEC primarily for the drug trade and the medical profession without the expectation of its entering a food product. In fact, this company will not be responsible to anyone so using FEC and thereby getting into trouble."[39]

When anticocaine publicity coincided with the disappearance of countless packaged remedies, reformers assumed that the education of the public had been the cause. One of the central elements of Progressive Era reform thought was the conceptualization of the consumer as a dupe, waiting to be exploited by corporate interests. Subsequent generations have been led to assert much the same thing; one historian, for example, argued that "drugs containing alcohol and narcotics were effectively eliminated when consumers were informed of their presence on the label."[40] To some extent, this observation holds true for products such as Maltine Coca Wine. What this view fails to consider is the extent to which the drug industry conceded the cocaine issue to the control interests. Ethical firms no longer regarded cocaine as centrally important to their business, whereas larger patent medicine firms sought to protect their other lines of consumer products. Also missing from the consumer-as-dupe model are those companies that resisted the control of their products and whose customers knew full well the nature of the drug they consumed.

The Resisters:
Nathan Tucker and the Failures of Regulation

Although the AMA and the Bureau of Chemistry were remarkably zealous in their pursuit of coca wines, soft drinks, and low-potency medications, they did not ignore the more potent catarrh cures. Indeed, as far back as the 1890s, commentators had identified the catarrh cures and cocaine snuffs as the most problematic of the forms available to the consumers. In 1897, the *Practical Druggist* published a formula for a "harmless catarrh cure" which designated as "harmful" any cure that contained cocaine.[41] The popular asthma and catarrh cures were targets of concerted efforts at legal control in the early 1900s. The federal government took action against all of the major products, including Az-Ma-Syde, Tucker's Asthma Specific, and E. H. Ryno's Hay Fever Cure. The popular press also targeted catarrh and asthma cures. Muckraking journalists such as Adams attacked the manufacturers of catarrh cures as "deliberate slayers of men's souls." For the maker of Birney's Catarrh Cure, Adams had nothing but contempt, writing that "there is in the whole United States no city whose God's acre does not hold the bones of his victims; whose jail records are not black with their crimes."[42]

What worried reformers the most was the link between the catarrh cures and the drug-taking culture of cocaine fiends. According to the *Midland Druggist* in 1903, "one of the chief causes of the cocaine habit is traceable directly to the use of secret preparations for catarrh which contain more or less of that drug."[43] In January 1917, Charles B. Towns, writing in the *Pharmaceutical Era,* looked back on the time of the peak use of cocaine and noted that "the horrible spread and use of cocaine grew out of the so-called catarrh cures, which contained from three to five percent of the drug. This quantity was supposed to be harmless, but every druggist knows how the sale of these 'catarrh cures' grew enormously merely on the strength of its cocaine content." The identities of these cures became so linked in the public mind with a certain product that a mixture of cocaine and lactose sold on the streets of New Orleans was popularly known as *crown* — the brand name of the product of the Crown Catarrhal Powder Company. When the Louisiana legislature eventually passed an anticocaine law, it prohibited both cocaine and crown.[44]

Unlike a great many drug manufacturers, the firms that produced the catarrh cures made only that one product. Moreover, the cocaine content of this product was well known; indeed, cocaine was their raison d'être. These firms were consequently not inclined to withdraw their only product under pressure from anticocaine publicity. Many such manufacturers openly defied what Charles L. Mitchell, maker of Coca-Bola, called "crank legislation." Because the cocaine content of these products was already well known, laws that mandated labeling — even state poison labels — had relatively less impact on such products.

Dr. Cole's Catarrh Cure and Dr. Birney's Catarrh Cure both appeared in 1907 with new de-cocainized versions, but the "cocainized" Cole's stayed on the market. Although Cole's manufacturer touted the new product as one that "cannot give rise to any so-called 'habit' in child or adult," they defiantly asserted that they did not "propose to give up the manufacture" of the original product, and "its manufacture and sale will be continued as heretofore." Consumers certainly knew the difference; druggists in New York faced angry customers who had purchased the new Birney's cure only to find that "these new ones don't do any good."[45]

Chief among the resisters was Dr. Nathan Tucker, the maker of Tucker's Asthma Specific, who defied the federal government for years. In a meeting with Harvey Wiley, Tucker's attorney challenged the notion that the labeling of his client's product as a "specific" for asthma constituted mislabeling. "If you will send out and bring in twenty-five of the worst cases of asthma," the attorney challenged Wiley, "I will demonstrate that it is a specific for asthma, and within three minutes from the time of application there will be an absolute and instantaneous relief of each and every one and I do not care of how long standing." Wiley commented sarcastically that "so good a thing ought to be widely published in medical journals." In fact, Tucker persisted in selling his product well into the 1920s, simply by complying with the labeling provisions of the Pure Food and Drug Act. Records of the Bureau of Narcotics indicate that Tucker's use of cocaine in production during 1926, for example, was as high as it had been fifteen years earlier. For Tucker, the efforts at regulation had little effect other than allowing consumers to determine more easily the relative strength of the available cocaine cures by requiring the contents to be labeled.[46]

Control advocates such as Adams recognized the failure of drug laws to limit the activities of manufacturers like Tucker. For cocaine habitués, he wrote, labeling provisions only "help them by giving information as to which nostrum is the most heavily drugged." In the words of a druggist, "when I see a customer comparing labels I know she's a fiend."[47]

Another conspicuous failure of regulation was the control of cocaine manufacture. Fewer than a dozen large chemical and pharmaceutical firms had supplied the drug industry with the cocaine needed to manufacture everything from corn cures to catarrh snuffs, and all were relatively insulated from the public furor over cocaine sales. Although the Pure Food and Drug Act restricted the use of cocaine in packaged remedies, it said nothing about the sale of cocaine itself. Indeed, as long as the cocaine met agreed-upon standards for purity and was labeled properly, there were no federal restrictions on its sale. Even the Harrison Act kept the focus on control of the retail distribution of cocaine, leaving untouched the chemical manufacturer of it. Not until passage of the Jones-Miller Act in 1922 did the federal government enact any serious restrictions on cocaine production.

To be sure, chemical companies such as the Mallinckrodt Chemical Works were as sensitive as any patent medicine maker when negative publicity threatened to intrude. In summer 1909, company executives screened a film entitled "The Curse of Cocaine." Produced by the Chicago-based Essanay Film Company, the film contained "nothing objectionable" as far as the executives were concerned except for one scene with a tight shot of a bottle of cocaine. In that shot, the company complained, the Mallinckrodt label was "made quite a prominent feature, as it is thrown on the screens separately in very much enlarged size so as to show clearly all of the printed matter on the label." Mallinckrodt requested that the offending image be deleted from the film, and although the company was slow to respond, the threat of legal action eventually produced the desired result. For the chemical industry, however, the threat of poor publicity rarely intruded upon its operations.[48]

In the meantime, pharmaceutical and chemical companies that produced cocaine do not appear to have diminished their total output of the drug despite the reduction in legal outlets for its sale. In the absence of any legal requirement that they do so, there was apparently little interest in limiting production voluntarily. The quantities of legally produced cocaine did decline over time but not nearly as rapidly as the number of legal outlets for its sale.

In the end, the legacies of the "propaganda for reform," as the AMA fashioned it, were decidedly mixed. It seems clear that the emergence of a coalition for cocaine control must have accomplished a dramatic reduction in the prevalence of cocaine consumption, as countless American consumers were offered new decocainized forms of popular products such as Vin Mariani and Coca-Cola. In response, most of these consumers appear to have simply abandoned their use of cocaine; certainly there is no evidence that these persons subsequently adopted the use of the pure cocaine that was still available. In the case of Coca-Cola and the soft drinks, the caffeine content (already present) provided a suitable stimulant effect. Because purchasers of Celery-Cola, Maltine, and other dilute oral dosage forms of cocaine accounted for a small share of overall cocaine sales, it is not surprising that general levels of cocaine consumption did not decline nearly as rapidly. On the contrary, cocaine consumption was still at its peak level as late as 1910 and may not have dropped off substantially until after 1920, by which time most cocaine preparations had already been removed from the market for several years. The market that remained was dominated by sales of pure cocaine, most of which went directly to the public through an increasingly marginalized network of distribution.

The great failure of the reformers was in making little distinction (pharmacological or otherwise) among various cocaine products or between cocaine and the coca leaf from which it came. Faced with a vast array of products and forms in which cocaine appeared, reformers sought to restrict access to them all. In the process, legitimate concerns over public health and illegitimate advertising were too often blended with imaginary fears and misleading generalizations.

This approach had a disastrous consequence for cocaine control because it helped demolish a thriving coca business that presented no great threat to public health while leaving cocaine production virtually untouched. By driving low-potency cocaine products off the market entirely, the field was left wide open to the sale of pure cocaine. Why was the focus off the mark? It may have been, as some have suggested, attributable to ignorance over the differences among various forms of cocaine and coca. Or it may have been, as some claimed at the time, that the control of cocaine could not have been accomplished without restricting all of its forms, including the coca leaf. But ignorance and expediency are only small parts of the answer. The effort at regulation reflected a dual impulse: one grounded in a concern for limiting the misuse of cocaine, the other in a desire to control the drug industry more generally. By the standards of the latter interest, no exceptions were possible; any commercial interest in cocaine would inevitably threaten the public interest if not the public health.

EIGHT

Consumers' Paradise?

A Shadow Market Emerges

Clerks often sold cocaine, but rarely mentioned it, in the Baltimore drugstores of Adam Huthwelker and Charles Sonnenberg. Located near one another in the city's western district, the two stores received a steady stream of regular customers seeking the drug. Entering the stores, would-be purchasers asked for "a trip to heaven," with "a return ticket" if the dose was to be doubled. Other frequent customers asked for "a box" or "a nail" when they entered. The clerks knew the code and used it themselves. Customers looking for boxes and nails would be asked, "how far do you want to go?" — the correct answer being "one block" or "two blocks" depending on the dose they sought.

The most interesting aspect of all of this activity is that the descriptions date from 1904, ten years before federal prohibition in the form of the Harrison Act. The practices of these two drugstores, repeated across the country, seem to defy traditional understanding of drug selling. The standard history of the drug trade features two "typical" types. The legal-era retailer is portrayed as a neighborhood druggist, supplying consumer demands for a safe and reliable product and assuring all consumers equal access to cocaine. The postprohibition drug dealer, on the other hand, generally appears as an uneducated peddler of drugs, preying upon customers, forcing prices up and product quality and safety down in the search for profit.[1]

The primary failing of this model is its inadequate explanation of the transformation itself. How exactly did this dramatic change in cocaine retailing take place? Was it sudden or gradual? How closely connected with cocaine prohibition were these changes? Huthwelker and Sonnenberg were hardly street peddlers, but they were also clearly operating in the shadows of legitimate business. Few studies address these questions; that the transformation occurred and that it occurred because of prohibition remain mainly articles of faith.

Finding better answers to these questions requires examination of the transactions between customer and retailer. Every drugstore sold some amount of cocaine, but what exactly did *selling cocaine* mean? Consumers entering a drugstore to purchase cocaine had to do more than simply buy the drug over the counter. Purchases would have to be justified to the druggist, who could refuse any particular sale. This discretionary power over drug sales became increasingly important as retail druggists defined the limits of legitimate cocaine selling. Some limitations were imposed on sellers externally either by informal community pressure or by formal regulations that sought to enforce the legitimate/illegitimate distinction. But many druggists were willing partners in drug control, accepting the negative view of cocaine and its users and employing participation in the control movement to assert claims of professional authority.

As many legal sources of supply imposed these limitations, a new network of sellers met consumer demand. Huthwelker's and Sonnenberg's drugstores were part of this network. As their counterparts in the Maryland and Baltimore druggists' associations traveled to Annapolis to lobby for anticocaine laws, these druggists showed their willingness to operate outside the boundaries of legitimate selling. The boundaries were still partly informal, so such sales did not, strictly speaking, constitute an illicit enterprise. The new enterprise might better be described as a *shadow market,* operating just beyond the edge of legitimate supply. Although not entirely satisfactory, the term highlights the gray area of cocaine selling. The shadow market made a direct connection to an emerging drug culture and took on features more closely associated with the illicit market of the 1920s and beyond.[2] Edward Brecher famously characterized the late nineteenth century as a kind of dope fiend's paradise in which drug users escaped the harms associated with illegal supply and in so doing avoided social sanction. Closer examination of the shadow market suggests, however, that for many cocaine users, the consumers' paradise never existed.

Caveat Vendor: The Limits of the Legal Supply

Retailers shouldered most of the blame for local cocaine problems. Early efforts at local control worked to define legitimate retail sales in much the same manner as the national reform coalition sought to restrict the illegitimate use of cocaine in pharmaceutical manufacturing. The concept of *illegitimate* retailing covered sales of cocaine outside the bounds of approved medical practice. The worst were those made to cocaine fiends or involving exceptionally large quantities. Any sale of cocaine which failed these informal tests was illegitimate although not necessarily illegal; the emerging standard of ethical cocaine selling had less to do with legality than it did with nascent efforts to establish professional norms.

As the popular use of cocaine grew, so too did the estimates of the proportion of cocaine which went to illegitimate use — most still dispensed, however, within existing legal standards. The most conservative of estimates, made by the head of one of the largest pharmaceutical firms in the United States in an effort to downplay the problem, conceded that "at least 20 percent is used for indulgence." At the other end of the estimate spectrum, anticocaine reformers had as large a stake in overstating the problem as the drug industry had in understatement. The police commissioner of New York City argued that "not less than 50 percent of the total sales of cocaine are for illegitimate purposes, and we believe that this estimate is far below the facts."[3] A key figure in this group, addiction specialist T. D. Crothers, claimed that only 3 to 8 percent of cocaine sales could be "accounted for in legitimate ways."[4]

The close relationship between retailer and consumer led, perhaps inevitably, to the identification of druggists with the spread and encouragement of nonmedical cocaine consumption. Drug manufacturers and physicians encouraged this view, blaming druggists for the diversion of cocaine to nonmedical purposes. As the secretary of the Medical Society of the County of New York described it, the role physicians recast for themselves was that of "protection of the simple minded and easily duped from the wiles of the drug charlatan."[5] With considerable success, manufacturers argued that keeping track of how the public used this product was neither possible nor was it their responsibility. Edward Mallinckrodt professed to be anxious to aid the government antinarcotic efforts but claimed that the "so-called 'fiends' are not supplied by manufacturers . . . but by unscrupulous retail druggists and other retail dealers and, to some extent, by unscrupulous physicians." Mallinckrodt urged the government to consider making nonprescription retail sales a "severely punishable" criminal offense because measures aimed at manufacturers would "in no wise prevent 'fiends' from getting all the 'dope' they are able to pay for or in any way restrict retail druggists."[6]

The association of druggists with the cocaine problem was not simply a matter of blame shifting by manufacturers and physicians. Many reformers saw control of retail distribution as the most promising strategy for dealing with nonmedical use. The anticocaine movement in Chicago, centered on Hull House, attacked the selling practices of the city's retail druggists, especially those on the West Side who supplied cocaine to teenagers living in the surrounding neighborhoods.[7] Jane Addams recalled that "the attempt on the part of Hull House residents to prohibit the sale of cocaine to minors" brought the settlement house "into sharp conflict with many druggists" who "only felt outraged and abused."[8]

The Hull House crusaders, like their reform-minded contemporaries, rarely mentioned drug manufacturers or wholesale firms. Instead, organizations as diverse as the New England Watch and Ward Society, the Henry Street Settlement, and the Women's Christian Temperance Union accused drugstores of serving as the headquarters for the degradation and ruin of American youth.

The cumulative effect of such criticisms was to strengthen the informal public pressure on druggists to conform to nascent standards of ethical selling — standards that often ran ahead of legal requirements. Indeed, the popular Progressive magazine, the *Independent,* editorialized that "it is the character of the druggist, however, much more than the legal regulations in the matter, that count for reform." Following this logic, the editorial continued, "when it is known that a particular druggist is careless in the matter of providing drugs for drug habitués then honest people should avoid him." If a sense of professional responsibility failed to prevent such sales, then a community might justifiably impose its own standards. The editorial concluded that this "may seem a very indirect way of combating so serious an evil, but it can be made very effective."[9]

State and local governments made many efforts to translate these informal public standards into formal controls. Indeed, more states and territories specifically regulated the sale of cocaine than any other drug, including morphine and heroin.[10] The earliest regulatory efforts were local, as cities with large cocaine markets sought to control sales. In New Orleans, a city ordinance did not prohibit the sale of cocaine or medicines containing cocaine in "recognized therapeutic doses" but did ban any preparations in which "the ingredient cocaine gives such proportions as to make its deliriant, or intoxicating, effect the main reason for their use." The ordinance was clearly intended to distinguish between legitimate and illegitimate forms of cocaine selling. Its primary failing was the lack of specificity about what exactly separated legitimate sale from illegitimate, a confusion that defendants sought to exploit in court.[11]

Other regulations targeted illegitimate sales with more specific requirements. These regulations usually prohibited certain forms of cocaine or its sale in large amounts. In 1913, the New York State legislature passed the Delahanty measure, which restricted the stocks of druggists to only 5 ounces at a time. The law also banned the sale of flake or crystal cocaine, used for cocaine sniffing. It did not restrict the sale of large crystal cocaine, used in the preparation of cocaine solutions — the form of cocaine used in medical and dental practice.[12] Another New York proposal, the Walker Anti-Cocaine Bill, which was strongly opposed by the drug lobby, confined druggists to a stock of no more than 1 ounce at a time and limited the sale of cocaine in solution to 4 percent, which was the strength most common in the use of it as an anesthetic.

In their effort to regulate the retail sale of cocaine, governments took a wide variety of approaches. Louisiana state law required retailers to "make affidavit that the drugs are for use in and sufficient for their legitimate trade" and that no cocaine be supplied to "any habitual user."[13] A provision in the 1905 Chicago Anti-Cocaine Ordinance required cocaine to be sold in packages no smaller than the smallest of original packages sold by wholesalers (1/8 ounce). This measure was designed to "stop the sale of cocaine and morphine for other than legitimate purposes," as the *Pharmaceutical Era* reported.[14]

Definitions of *illegitimate* selling also influenced the punishments accorded cocaine law violators. Druggists who violated regulations received sentences that varied according to both the perceived seriousness of the offense and the character of the offender. When a spectacular 1910 raid in Pittsburgh rounded up more than sixty druggists and clerks, variations in their treatment revealed much about the *intent* of regulation. Judge Marshall Brown imposed a fine on those pharmacists "otherwise doing a legitimate business" (represented by a lawyer from the Western Pennsylvania Retail Druggists Association [WPRDA]) and warned them not to remain ignorant of state laws. Pharmacists selling cocaine to peddlers or who sold to fiends were sent to the city workhouse.[15] Not long after this incident, the WPRDA journal reported the arrest of an illegitimate cocaine seller: "A foreigner with an unpronounceable name conducting, or at least pretending to do so, an alleged pharmacy at Duquesne, was up before the court a few days since to answer to the charge of selling Cocaine to a boy, and with soliciting sales through agents." The Duquesne druggist's sales practices appear to have been illegitimate, yet the attitude of the WPRDA clearly reflected its bias against a foreign druggist in a working-class mill town (who, additionally, did not belong to the WPRDA). When the druggist received only two months in jail and a $100 fine, the journal expressed its dismay at the lenient treatment.[16]

The response of druggists to regulatory efforts exposed tensions within retail pharmacy. Defensively, druggists attempted to shift the blame elsewhere. Even the most prestigious of pharmacy organizations, the American Pharmaceutical Association (APhA), was led to complain that "when a manufacturer or jobber supplies a small retail drugstore with pounds of morphine and cocaine every month, can it be said that they do not know the reason for such unusual orders?" Before punishing "the little fellows," said the APhA, policy makers should look "higher up" to the sources of cocaine.[17]

Druggists also invoked their traditional right to sell whatever drug they wished to customers, especially when faced with food and drug legislation intended to restrict the sales of specific products.[18] One druggist, responding to criticism that he had sold cocaine to a notorious fiend, observed, "We try to discourage people who take cocaine. When a beginner comes in and asks for it we discourage him, but a man like Wilson must have it."[19] Protests over investigative tactics further exposed the conflict between traditional discretion and modern regulation. Druggists took particular offense at undercover "sting" operations. Typically, investigators would enter a drugstore, requesting cocaine and citing urgent medical need. When inspectors in New York began fining druggists who provided the cocaine, one professional journal complained that "while it is true that indiscriminate cocaine sellers should be prosecuted, still it does seem as though less trickery on the part of the inspectors is desirable."[20]

On the other hand, many retail druggists used that same discretion to limit cocaine sales voluntarily. The cautions against the free use of cocaine by the lay public which filled the editorial pages of national medical journals found a place in the pharmaceutical press as well. From the druggists' perspective, catarrh cures highlighted all of the most uncomfortable issues involving cocaine selling. Not only were the inexpensive and prepackaged powders closely identified with non-medical consumption and the stereotypical cocaine fiend, but their popularity left druggists vulnerable to the accusation that they merely vended patent medicine without exercising reasonable professional caution.

Voluntary cooperation in restricting sales seemed to be a viable alternative to legal controls. As early as 1894, the *Druggists' Circular* had warned its readership of the dangers posed by the easy distribution of Birney's Catarrh Cure. By the turn of century, the rhetoric of the retail drug trade grew stronger along with the anticocaine movement. The *Midland Druggist,* an Ohio pharmaceutical journal, urged the state's druggists to check the cocaine "evil" by discarding all questionable catarrh cures and to inform all customers inquiring after such products of the reasons they were no longer available. To those concerned over discontinuing a popular product, the journal reassuringly argued that customers would "thank" such a retailer and "remember him for his honesty . . . This would be a step in the right direction," the journal concluded, "the beginning of the wedge which is destined to lay open the secrets of the peoples' murderers."[21]

As the language of the *Midland Druggist* suggests, professionally minded druggists embraced the reformers' message.[22] This acceptance of the anticocaine message, as much as professional self-interest, influenced druggists on both an individual and an organizational level. If, as the *American Druggist* suggested, the creation of pharmacy laws had established "to a certain extent a privileged class [of retailers] to whom alone is extended the privilege of dealing in drugs and poisons," the privilege carried a "corresponding degree of responsibility."[23] The editorial posture of the *National Druggist,* a conservative journal based in St.

Louis, is interesting in this regard. A fierce opponent of all food and drug laws, the journal ridiculed the goals of drug regulation and engaged in regular attacks on Harvey Wiley, Samuel Hopkins Adams, and the leadership of the American Medical Association. Yet this same journal, where cocaine selling was concerned, urged that "the retail druggists themselves be the first to expose the misdoings of their associates and to see that the perpetrators are brought to justice."[24]

Even Samuel Hopkins Adams, so often a critic of the drug business, conceded the impact of voluntary sales restrictions. If catarrh cures such as Birney's and Agnew's were now "at the end of their rope," Adams observed, this could be attributed to the actions of retail druggists as much as the impact of food and drug legislation: "In store after store of the better class, my inquiries for the catarrh snuffs have been met with the curt rejoinder: 'No you can't buy that rotten stuff here.'"[25] Adams claimed to have visited twenty pharmacies in New York State and obtained cocaine at only one. He noted approvingly a Chicago druggist who had his catarrh cures analyzed after observing how "shop girls from a great department store" frequently stopped to purchase them at noon. After learning they contained cocaine, he discarded his remaining stock. Even granting Adams' penchant for hyperbole and exaggeration, some pharmacists clearly exercised their authority to refuse to dispense cocaine and cocaine-based products.

Joining the cocaine control forces not only afforded druggists an opportunity to reinforce their claims to professional status, it also allowed them to influence the content and direction of any new legislation.[26] One pharmaceutical publication made the case directly: "the public is not in position to judge who the violators are. Let the druggists exert their influence and with the help of the citizenship bring these transgressors to justice . . . the moral qualifications are quite as essential as the educational of those who should be licensed as pharmacists."[27] James H. Beal of the APhA argued that "if the druggists of the United States do not resolutely take hold of the regulation of the sale of narcotic drugs . . . they will merely be turning it over to the care of people who are less competent to deal with it than themselves."[28]

After the Civil War, many states established state pharmacy boards to oversee the implementation of educational and licensing requirements for drug sellers. This existing regulatory structure proved a useful legal foundation for control over cocaine distribution; state pharmacy boards often held or shared responsibility for enforcement of state cocaine laws.[29] In Pennsylvania, the Board of Pharmacy and its crusading vice president, Dr. Christopher Koch Jr., investigated charges of excessive cocaine selling in Philadelphia and Pittsburgh. Based on the results of personal investigations by Koch and his counsel, Samuel Clement Jr., the board conducted a drug sweep in Philadelphia which netted more than sixty people. Of those arrested, about a dozen were retail druggists, and another dozen were drug clerks.[30]

Using state authority to control the licensing of pharmacists, the Kentucky Board of Pharmacy waged an impressive war against druggists who sold cocaine, stripping several of their licenses. Like many of the anticocaine statutes, regulations embedded within state pharmacy laws targeted illegitimate sales, a concept that could never be defined with precision. The Kentucky pharmacy code prohibited the sale of cocaine for "illegitimate purposes" but failed to define exactly what those were. When Henry Cohn, a Louisville pharmacist, had his license to practice revoked for illegitimate cocaine sales, he unsuccessfully appealed on the grounds that the rules provided no definition of *illegitimate*.[31] In Cleveland, the local druggists association suspended cocaine sellers from its membership only by using a clause in its rules which permitted the suspension of members for "gross immorality." According to the secretary of the State Board of Pharmacy, "such action would have more effect in suppressing the cocaine traffic than almost any other plan that could be devised."[32]

The Illinois State Board of Pharmacy took the additional step of becoming an active member of the anticocaine effort. Starting in 1904, in an effort to prevent sales of cocaine to minors, the state board joined Hull House, Chicago's juvenile court committee, and the Legal Aid Society in conducting investigations and seeking prosecutions under authority of state drug laws. In a letter to twenty-five druggists under investigation, the board warned them against selling cocaine without a prescription. Should a recipient of this letter continue to violate state drug laws, "you, and you alone, are responsible for the trouble that comes to you."[33] Here was the most explicit statement yet that professional pharmacy, on the question of cocaine control, would side with the forces of control against individual pharmacists' traditional liberties.

Origins of the Shadow Market

Informal limits on legitimate cocaine selling combined with the imposition of some formal regulations created an environment in which the legitimate market was either unwilling or unable to supply the demands of recreational users. In this climate, alternative sources of supply which were clearly illegitimate, if not actually illegal, sprang up to meet an unsatisfied demand. As further encouragement, cocaine selling presented opportunities for remarkable profit because many consumers had little choice but to pay a premium for the dealer's readiness to meet all requests for cocaine.

The appearance of a shadow market shows access to cocaine in the preprohibition era to have been more difficult than previously thought. As the only source of cocaine for many poor and working-class consumers, the underground market preyed easily on those who depended on its supply. Many features associated with the subsequent illicit market of the post–Harrison Act era, especially inflated retail prices, characterized the underground market as well. The similarities are striking enough to demonstrate that drug prohibition alone did not create the hostile, dangerous, and costly drug-using environment characteristic of much of the twentieth century.

The New Cocaine Entrepreneurs

The formal and informal measures that led numerous druggists to discard their catarrh cures did not, at least immediately, make much impact on cocaine consumption. Reflecting a fairly steady demand for the drug, the legal manufacture and importation of cocaine did not begin to decline until after 1910 (and then only gradually). In the interim, a new group of retailers embraced cocaine selling as a primary occupation, stepping in where legitimate sources of supply fell short. These new sellers included doctors and druggists as well as peddlers with little or no connection to the legal drug distribution system. Collectively, they created a new marketplace for cocaine and added to the range of underground enterprises.

At the very top of the shadow network were retail druggists for whom cocaine selling became a primary, even exclusive, function. Although the concept of underground sales was imprecise and carried various levels of meaning, an underground seller might be identified by that most basic measure of practice, volume of sales. Estimates of the quantity of cocaine which might be distributed as part of *legitimate* drugstore business varied a good deal, of course, depending on who was making the estimate. On the high end, the police commissioner of New York City estimated that "a large drugstore" would sell about 1 to 3 ounces of cocaine a month "for legitimate purposes."[34] At the lower end of the scale, a correspondent to the *Pharmaceutical Era* felt that "a pharmacist in the legitimate use of the drug handles only 2 ounces a year."[35] One city might produce very different versions of what constituted legitimate selling practice. In New Orleans, the district attorney investigating cocaine selling concluded that the city's 190 drugstores ought not to consume more than 100 to 150 ounces per year. Yet the text of a New Orleans grand jury report made public at the same time offered as acceptable the more liberal allowance of 1 ounce per month in each drugstore. With 190 drugstores, the higher figure amounted to 2,280 ounces annually — giving two quite different "legitimate" totals for New Orleans!

What these disparities cannot hide, however, is that actual cocaine sales in cities around the United States dwarfed even the most generous estimates of legitimate trade. In New Orleans, local wholesalers sold at least 3,500 to 4,000 ounces of pure cocaine to city druggists in a ten-month period; nor was this the only cocaine sold in New Orleans, for druggists also ordered cocaine from drug wholesalers in St. Louis, Chicago, and elsewhere. Cocaine sales in the city were therefore at least twice as high as the most liberal estimate of legitimate cocaine consumption.[36]

A small number of drugstores dominated the city's cocaine trade. Aaron Martin was among the most prominent of these. Martin owned a 6-foot by 8-foot drugstore, with an inventory (cocaine excluded) worth no more than $100. Yet Martin purchased 470 ounces of cocaine from one wholesale drug dealer in just nine months.[37] Valuing each ounce of cocaine at the wholesale price of $3, Martin had purchased more than $1,400 worth of cocaine. Even at legitimate retail prices, Martin's cocaine had a resale value of more than $4,000, a sum equivalent to the entire annual sales of many of the city's largest drugstores.[38]

In Pittsburgh, a 1903 estimate of consumption by the state pharmaceutical board suggested that druggists sold a combined total of 300 ounces per month. One owner of a downtown drugstore related that he personally sold 40 to 50 ounces of cocaine per month, about 15 percent of the city's total. After surveying cocaine selling in Pittsburgh, Thomas Simonton concluded that although some druggists refused to dispense cocaine except on prescription and even refused to carry cocaine-based catarrh cures, a minority of drugstores supplied most cocaine: "it is the honest belief of this writer that three thousand ounces, or 1,440,000 grains, is not an unusual amount to pass over a single counter in a year, but actual figures are hard to obtain."[39] Simonton failed to document his claim of 3,000 ounces, but his evidence shows that the bulk of the Pittsburgh cocaine supply, like that of New Orleans, was controlled by relatively few druggists.

Individual druggists like Adolph Brendecke of Chicago, the "chief of cocaine sellers," acquired substantial reputations for their role in the trade.[40] Brendecke did business from his South Side drugstore, combining wholesale and retail functions. Although Brendecke sold directly to consumers, most of his business depended upon sales to so-called *peddlers* of cocaine, a term that applied very generally to any sellers who were not doctors or druggists.[41]

The most prominent cocaine peddlers purchased large quantities of it from druggists like Brendecke or diverted supplies from wholesalers and manufacturers.[42] In Chicago, the most famous of the peddlers was Eugene Hustion, an African-American cocaine distributor in the city's South Side levee district. Hustion and his college-educated wife Lottie began their operations in 1904 and were still selling cocaine in 1914. The Hustions obtained their supply through the wholesale drug firm of Knox, Greene & Company, operated several "subagencies" throughout the South Side, stocked more than 30 pounds of cocaine at their Dearborn Street location, and sent runners nightly to some of the most famous houses of prostitution in the city. According to Hustion, he had "gross daily sales as high as $200, of which $160 was profit."[43]

Although druggists like Brendecke and peddlers like Hustion controlled much of the Chicago underground cocaine trade, highly centralized distribution networks similar to those of the postprohibition era were rarely seen in Chicago or elsewhere. Instead, the evidence seems substantially to confirm one analyst's observations about the decentralized nature of cocaine distribution in New York City during the 1910s. Many dealers continued to operate independently or in conjunction with one or two other dealers. None of the retailing combinations was especially large; certainly none was large enough or important enough to dominate the market for cocaine in the city.[44]

The position of the cocaine peddler was almost certainly strengthened by the manner in which cities and states regulated cocaine sales. In one instance of inadvertent support for peddlers, the widespread drugstore sales of cocaine in small packages costing 10¢ and 15¢ led Chicago to set a minimum amount of cocaine for each transaction. The intent of the regulation was to discourage consumers by making drugstore purchases of cocaine more costly. Instead, the effort almost certainly accelerated the emergence of peddlers who purchased the larger amounts and then resold the drug in smaller quantities.

The widespread absence of laws against the possession of cocaine also proved to be a benefit to peddlers.[45] In most instances, for a violation of state or local law to have occurred, a peddler had to be caught in the process of selling the drug. These requirements made enforcement efforts aimed at peddlers more difficult than regulation of druggists operating from fixed locations.[46] Prosecutors in Galveston, Texas, complained that "we have several dives here operating through sale of drugs but we cannot get the evidence of sale even when our officers seize the drug as it is not against the law for one not a druggist to have the drug in his possession, and the law ought to be that one not a druggist who has over a certain quantity in possession is guilty, and no proof of sale required."[47] The *Outlook* noted gloomily that "in Chicago the Hull House managers tried over and over again to convict these 'runners,' or street peddlers; but although they could easily arrest them with packages of cocaine on their persons, it was impossible to obtain a conviction unless actual sale was proven." After the arrest of George Dillon and William Wolff, caught in their New York apartment with several bottles of cocaine, the presiding judge ordered the two released, ruling that "it was no crime to have cocaine in one's possession."[48]

Independent peddlers included both those who sold cocaine as a full-time occupation and those who merely supplemented other kinds of income. The more substantial peddlers often employed fixed locations, such as the residents of a Brooklyn tenement raided in 1911, in the possession of "one four-pound bottle of flake cocaine, two two-pound bottles, ninety-five smaller bottles, and eighteen boxes of the contraband drug," all hidden beneath a trapdoor in the third floor.[49] Leading peddlers in Pittsburgh obtained their cocaine in 7-pound jars from out-of-town druggists (apparently less inclined to ask questions).[50]

Small-time retailers tended to select as their fixed locations street corners or hotel rooms. Most often, they simply carried their stock of cocaine with them. Harris Dickson, writing to Hamilton Wright, claimed that cocaine "can be easily peddled about and sold from the pocket of a vagrant negro—man or woman—who passes amongst the camps, railroads and other places where negroes are employed."[51] The highly public nature of their business exposed this level of sellers to a greater risk of police harassment or arrest as Virginia Telfrey could readily attest after her fourth arrest in New Orleans, the last with two cigar boxes full of cocaine in her possession, prepared in packages selling for 15¢, 25¢, and 50¢.[52]

The operations of full-time dealers required numerous part-time employees to carry out various functions. Some druggists employed runners to create a market outside of their stores and to minimize their risk of disruption at the same time. Runners also directed or steered customers to the druggist's location. The Vice Commission of Chicago observed that "there are four druggists whose method of catering to prostitutes is to send clerks to their respective customers in the various houses of prostitution to solicit orders." Other elements of the distribution network included messenger boys who were frequently employed by prostitutes to deliver cocaine from nearby drugstores. A district madam, according to the commission, "is in the habit of calling up Mr. —— and ordering a certain quantity of cocaine, who in turn calls this messenger boy and sends it out to her residence." In this way, "the messenger becomes an important link in the system whereby cocaine and various other drugs used by habitués are secured by them." On one such occasion, the messenger, "suspecting it was cocaine," sniffed some of the drug. The commission reported that "he stated that he had done this a considerable number of times since and seemed to have derived a good deal of pleasure out of it."[53] Another prostitute determined that messenger boys "talked too much and cannot be trusted" and instead commissioned a newsboy to purchase cocaine for her.[54]

The bottom of the underground distribution system included cocaine users who resold part of their purchases in order to maintain their habits. A 1920 account of San Francisco cocaine selling described how many users supported their habits through sales of cocaine. Writer Fred Williams reported that "eventually the majority of the dope addicts turn peddlers to obtain the money with which to buy their dope. They will buy a dram, cut it up into 'bindles,' reserve a few 'shots' for themselves and peddle the remainder." According to Williams, "there are more than 500 peddlers of dope in San Francisco when the dope addict who sells half his buy is taken into consideration."[55]

In an effort to increase profits and stretch scarce supplies, underground sellers usually reduced the purity of the cocaine they sold. Of course, catarrh cure manufacturers had long recognized the benefits of combining cocaine with other, cheaper ingredients that would provide bulk to the product at minimal cost. By mixing cocaine with an ingredient such as lactose, the retailer created a product that was palatable and profitable. Although lactose (often called sugar of milk) cost only pennies a pound, it was not the only product with which retailers adulterated their product. Early analgesics, such as acetanilide and phenacetin, were also commonly found in cocaine mixtures.[56] Even though these products were part of many proprietary remedies, in sufficient quantities they could be irritating or injurious to their consumers, particularly if the diluted mixtures were injected. In his account of the drug culture of San Francisco, Fred Williams claimed that "nine out of ten dope users have sores all over their bodies — due to the sugar of milk with which the drug is adulterated."[57]

As heavily adulterated cocaine, known as *crown* in New Orleans and *scrap* in Pittsburgh, came to dominate the underground supply, it became more expensive as well.[58] The New York City shadow market enjoyed an extraordinary profit margin. The amount of cocaine in a street deck selling for 25¢ was estimated as about 1.3 grains (85 milligrams), which translates into eleven times the wholesale price for cocaine. Price levels in other areas of the United States confirm that a shadow market developed under the legal, regulated market, raising the price of cocaine.

The trend toward higher prices actually began before 1900, with the rise in popular use. The New Orleans *Item*, for example, reported in 1900 the sales practices of a French Quarter druggist, Charles T. Simon, whose drugstore was "the central distribution point for cocaine fiends from all over the city." On the side of the drugstore, according to the newspaper account, was a door with one pane of glass broken out. At night, numerous customers would purchase cocaine through the hole in the door. Simon sold cocaine worth 1¢ to these nighttime purchasers for 5¢.[59]

Cocaine prices varied by location; certain groups of cocaine users had to bear the most substantial increases in price imposed by the underground sellers. The

Literary Digest outlined the cost of cocaine in New York City, providing a menu of prices which suggests that cocaine sniffers and the seriously habituated were left to bear the higher costs: "An ounce of cocain, wholesale, costs about $4. Divided into pink pill-boxes and blue bottles, the ounce is sold without adulteration for from $20 to $25 to those who use the needle and know the difference. Adulterated heavily with acetanilide it is sold to 'sniffers' for from $40 to $50 an ounce, and half-crazed fiends on the verge of the 'cocain leaps' can be made to yield an even greater profit."[60] That consumers readily paid these high prices is testimony to the shrinkage in the capacity of the legal market in the early twentieth century to supply the growing demands of nonmedical, recreational users and abusers of cocaine.

The Geography of the Shadow Market

In 1896, E. R. Waterhouse, a St. Louis physician, described a "cocaine joint disguised as a drugstore" operating in that city. His is one of the earliest publicized accounts of the cocaine underground (although the description tends to confuse the effects of cocaine and opium):

> This store had very well stocked shelves, but seldom was anything sold except cocaine; this was put up in packages which sold at a dime; after it was put up in the paper, it was rolled with a heavy iron roller to reduce the crystals to a powder. A pair of portiers covered a door back of the prescription counter, which was kept locked. The interior of this room was dark and contained chairs and two long benches. The cocaine fiend was admitted, and taking a seat, snuffed the powdered drug into the nose. A sort of dreamy intoxication followed, not unlike the Chinaman "hitting the pipe" in Dope Alley. A peep into the room, that was gotten through the strategy of a female reporter, disclosed the forms of a dozen or more, mostly of the lower class of prostitutes, black as well as white, upon the benches and floor. When they regained consciousness, should they desire more of the drug, they touched the bell, and in came the clerk with another dose, or should they be satisfied they stole quietly out the back door into the alley . . . The crowd which fills this man's coffers began coming as early as nine o'clock in the evening and at two or three o'clock in the night his room was full.[61]

Despite the obvious conflation of opium smoking and cocaine sniffing (it may be that both drugs were used in this "cocaine joint"), the report serves as a useful reminder of the importance of the physical settings to the trade. As the older legal market gradually faded away, the remaining underground sellers concentrated increasingly in specific geographic areas.

In cities, cocaine sales coexisted comfortably with the distribution of other illegitimate activities, such as gambling and prostitution. Consequently, city tenderloin districts and red-light areas came to be most closely associated with underground cocaine selling. As one study documents for Manhattan in the 1910s, sellers depended upon an urban network of institutions such as theaters, hotels, saloons, and newsstands.[62]

New York City, the center for legitimate cocaine importation, manufacture, and wholesale distribution, was also the home of a thriving shadow market. A police investigation of the cocaine trade in 1909 produced a list of sixty-three "suspicious" drugstores.[63] Much of the trade centered in the city's famous tenderloin district on Manhattan's West Side. Cocaine selling also reportedly had become a significant part of the underground economies of the Bowery and Chinatown.[64] On the northern fringe of the tenderloin, cocaine sellers flourished in the rapidly growing Times Square theater district.

Druggists in these areas, particularly in the tenderloin and Seventh Avenue, had been the source of smoking opium and morphine for years. In 1908, when Hamilton Wright solicited information about New York's opium problem, a number of respondents opined that cocaine "was rapidly taking the place of opium." A police officer stationed in the tenderloin for six years declared that "today cocaine tended to drive out the use of opiates, but that, in many cases, the use of the drugs was combined."[65] According to Samuel Hopkins Adams, the sale of catarrh cures for recreational use was so prevalent that "you may see the empty boxes and the instructive labels littering the gutters of Broadway any Saturday night." Indeed, one enterprising druggist in the area assembled a large window display consisting entirely of a large pyramid of boxes of Birney's cure.[66]

These urban neighborhoods housed not only the retail drugstores that supported the underground selling networks but also the many cocaine peddlers that coexisted with them. In New York "there were at least nine different types of place in and on which retailers conducted business: parks, drugstores, hotels, restaurants, saloons, pool parlors, theaters, public buildings, and certain street corners."[67] Frank McGuire, physician at the city prison, noted that "bartenders, night watchmen, and janitors" throughout the tenderloin provided users "tips" on where they might safely procure cocaine.[68]

The geography of cocaine selling in Pittsburgh illustrates the concentration of underground sales. The most prominent cocaine-selling district in the city was a small area adjacent to both downtown and the predominantly black Hill district. Tunnel Street, according to Thomas Simonton, was called "Cocaine Street" by its residents. The sociological study, the "Pittsburgh Survey," made the same observation. According to the survey, "there is much immorality in this section . . .

speakeasies, cocaine joints and disorderly houses abound." In January 1903, Simonton "procured a colored man" and instructed him to visit twelve drugstores in that part of Pittsburgh and attempt to purchase 15¢ worth of cocaine. At five of the twelve drugstores the man was refused because he did not have a prescription for the cocaine, reemphasizing the continuing reluctance of some druggists (even in areas where underground cocaine sales were substantial) to sell the drug. At six others, cocaine was forthcoming, "no questions being asked." According to Simonton, one druggist relocated his business from the area because cocaine sales had become too important to its health. Another druggist excused his cocaine sales by noting that his clerk had told him that if they did not sell it, "the trade would go somewhere else."[69]

The druggists of Chicago's levee district enjoyed what the *American Druggist* referred to as a "very lucrative" trade in cocaine. The Vice Commission of Chicago observed that although drugstores outside the levee district sold no more than 3 drams (3/8 ounce) of cocaine a month, stores within the vice district averaged at least 6 ounces of cocaine a month. Sellers also operated from other fixed locations throughout the levee, including hotels, saloons, brothels, cigar stores, newsstands, pool halls, private homes, apartments, street corners, and alleys. Despite the diversity of settings, long-time customers always seemed to know where and how to locate a seller. In the course of one hour in the summer of 1914, investigators from Charles Merriam's City Council Committee on Crime observed thirty-seven people "of all classes, both white and black" knock at the back door of one South Side residence and purchase small packages of cocaine. As the investigators noted, "some of the men and women could not wait until they got out of sight and snuffed the cocaine in the alley back of this place," where some of the users sat for hours drinking beer and sniffing cocaine, periodically going back to the building for more. Although such a system of distribution may have seemed wide open, it was closed in important ways—one investigator approached the back door three times without it opening, apparently being unaware of the correct knock.[70]

The experience of Merriam's investigator hints at a still more important defining characteristic of the underground cocaine trade: the networks of relationships between sellers and their customers. In general, sellers operated a distribution system closed to those without connections. The drug trade relied on trust and long-term relationships, a reciprocal arrangement in which sellers demanded the discretion and loyalty of buyers, and buyers rewarded those sellers with a reputation for providing a product of consistent quality and avoiding police entanglements.

Well before most formal regulation, the act of buying and selling cocaine took on qualities that revealed a tacit understanding between buyer and seller of the underground nature of the transaction. The language of buying and selling had its roots in an emerging drug culture that referred to cocaine as *coke, snow,* and *having a blow.* The consistency with which sellers employed these codes, however, highlights the functional purpose of concealing the nature of the transaction from either social or legal sanction.

Even in smaller towns, the location and appearance of a drugstore could signal the availability of cocaine. For most potential consumers, and particularly the less affluent, the larger and more prominent drugstores were less likely to supply their demand, and they consequently sought more marginal drugstores whose owners might have less concern for their professional standing as druggists. As a Vicksburg, Mississippi, attorney recounted to Hamilton Wright, "I do not believe as a rule that it [cocaine] is bought from reputable drugstores in any of the towns. I do not think these people handle cocaine at all. But there is a smaller class of semi-reputable drugstores who do handle it. I have myself known of strangers who wanted cocaine inquiring for a drugstore. When pointed out a big well-regulated drugstore they say "Not that kind. Isn't there a little one around the corner?"[71]

It has long been assumed that federal drug prohibition fundamentally altered the cocaine business. That assumption makes far too easy an equation between a drug's legal status, on the one hand, and its availability and social acceptability, on the other. Far from being able to ply their trade in peaceful obscurity because of the legal status of their business, cocaine retailers faced critical scrutiny from within their communities.

In a period of rising medical and social concerns (some real and some imagined) about unrestricted cocaine use, a definition of *legitimate selling* emerged from the anticocaine propaganda of reform groups and temperance organization and the endorsement of voluntary controls by professional pharmacy organizations. Countless individual druggists made the critical decision of whether to sell cocaine in limited ways or at all. This decision was not always based simply, or equitably, on the known dangers of cocaine; druggists claimed the right to refuse cocaine sales on the basis of the consumer's social status or race as well. The cumulative effect of these individual decisions was to close equal access to the legal supply of cocaine. This, in turn, became a powerful factor in the creation of the shadow market.

Conclusion

The Foundations of Modern Drug Control

Throughout the twentieth century, critics of national drug policy have decried the absence of "rationality" in drug control. Central to this critique is the assertion that American drug laws are the product of political imperatives, moralistic attitudes, and stereotypes of users which take little note of objective, scientific assessment of the relative harms of specific substances.[1] Moreover, critics charge that evaluating drugs by moral or political criteria leads to poor results or, as one notable critic of prohibition concluded, "a drug policy shaped by rhetoric and fear-mongering can only lead to our current disaster."[2] History supports their observation: legal prohibitions on opium, alcohol, cocaine, heroin, and marijuana were all advanced partly on the idea that their users were deviant, dangerous "others" whom no society could safely tolerate. Each substance was once a significant part of the therapeutic arsenal of "legitimate" medicine, and each was subsequently identified as "illegitimate" because of concerns that were at least as influenced by fear and prejudice as by objective evaluations of the harms they caused.

From this point of view, the introduction of rationality to policy making must involve a greater role for medical science and expert knowledge, as the numerous proposals for a "medicalization" of drug control attest. The earliest critics of American drug control shared this view, blaming the diminution of the physician's role in the distribution and control of opiates for the woeful state of the twentieth-century addict. For critics such as Alfred Lindesmith, the so-called British model, which allowed individual physicians to prescribe maintenance doses of opiates to addicts, usefully placed decision making in the hands of doctors.[3] Lindesmith explicitly raised the issue of providing a *legitimate* source of supply for addicts; his use of the term strongly suggests that he believed that legal sources of supply could not only eliminate the harms of the illicit market but could also reduce much of the stigma of addiction.[4]

In recent decades, reformers continue to echo the faith in physicians and science as a source of nonpolitical, rational drug laws, which a number of current examples make clear. In a 1996 article in the *Journal of the American Medical Association* (*JAMA*), Drs. Dorothy Hatusukami and Marian W. Fischman challenged the medical basis of federal sentencing guidelines for powder and crack cocaine. The authors argued that the physiological and psychoactive effects of the two substances were so similar that the large sentencing discrepancy (a 100:1 ratio) appeared "excessive." As Dr. Fischman noted, "the important issue is when possible to try and have science inform policy."[5] Debates over medical marijuana also raise the issue of privileging medical opinion over political or moral attitudes. In a 1995 *JAMA* editorial, Lester Grinspoon and James B. Bakalar pleaded that "it is time for physicians to acknowledge more openly that the present classification [of marijuana] is scientifically, legally, and morally wrong."[6]

As the search for alternatives to the current war on drugs has shifted somewhat from the British model of opiate maintenance to the Dutch model of "harm reduction," the arguments of reformers continue to stress the importance of judging drugs by objective standards. In a comprehensive harm reduction policy proposal that typifies the new objectivist approach, Avram Goldstein and Harold Kalant endorsed the utility of medical science as a nonpolitical basis for developing policy, using "the model of the FDA, whose mission, with respect to therapeutic agents, is to match the degree of regulation to the actual danger each presents." The authors conclude that "if removing the drug problem from politics is not yet feasible, the legislature should at least be guided . . . by the best factual information from non-government experts."[7]

The arguments for rational alternatives to contemporary drug policy provide a compelling counterpoint to the strident moralizing and punitive orientation of the current drug war. They make the promise of rational drug policy based on objective decision making quite explicit. They also invite a reconsideration of historical experience.

The Politics of Control

If ever a historical moment should have produced a coherent and rational approach to cocaine, it should have been in the years before legislatures began to regulate access. Physicians were the gateway to cocaine for most consumers, and doctors were free to follow their best professional judgments regarding appropriate prescription. The burgeoning field of pharmacological research promised to identify the risks and benefits of the physiological action of cocaine. Experimentation of all kinds went forward without interference from the state.

Indeed, the promise of rational decision making is evident everywhere during the medical era. One cannot help but be struck by the sophistication of doctors' treatment of cocaine, their attentiveness to the effects of form, dosage, route of administration, and even setting. The early medical literature reveals a remarkable degree of sensitivity to cocaine effects and a level of understanding which would be (sadly) unmatched until very recently. Even as physicians worried about cocaine poisoning and the cocaine habit, few doctors or pharmacists took an extreme position for or against cocaine. Even J. B. Mattison, who devoted much of his career to inveighing against the overuse of cocaine in medical practice, conceded that cocaine had uses as well as dangers and that the best approach would balance the potential harm with potential utility.[8]

Doctors took their role as gatekeeper to the drug supply seriously, avoiding indiscriminate prescription and paying attention to therapeutic outcomes. Some applications provided clear benefit, such as the use of cocaine to anesthetize the surface of the nasal mucosa. In other instances, purported benefits of cocaine turned out to be illusory, such as in the treatment of opiate addiction. Although initial reports suggested that cocaine might cure addiction, reports of disastrous outcomes brought a decisive turn in medical opinion.

The careful exercise of professional authority was, however, only one part of the cocaine experience. Equally important were the political dimensions of the "expert" role, made manifest through the actions of the medical/pharmaceutical practitioner and the institutional objectives of professional organizations. In its most basic form, the politics of professionalism generated a dual impulse: one grounded in a concern for limiting the harms associated with cocaine, the other in a desire to control the drug industry more generally.

This dual impulse exposes the compromises in modern drug control. Standards of legitimate cocaine use might incorporate clinical experience and laboratory research but also the belief that nonmedical distribution, promotion, and use were inappropriate per se. For individual doctors and druggists, cocaine appeared to be precisely the kind of drug that would prove dangerous in the hands of the general public. To keep the genie in the bottle meant self-regulation of the kind a Philadelphia physician practiced: "when it is necessary to prescribe a solution of cocaine for a patient to use himself within the nose, some precautions should be adopted to prevent him from forming the cocaine habit. It is well not to inform him of the name and nature of the drug given."[9] Alternatively, self-regulation could also mean keeping cocaine out of the hands of unreliable patients and customers.

The ability of drug makers to deliver cocaine directly to consumers merely redirected the control impulse from the individual level toward the organizational level. At this point, concerns over the popular use of cocaine effectively merged with a broader conflict over control of the nation's drug supply. Doctors, druggists, and even drug manufacturers recognized that active participation in cocaine control could reinforce claims to professional status and would allow them to influence the content and direction of new legislation.

Appreciating these interests explains an embrace of reform which otherwise would be hard to comprehend. Organizations of retail pharmacists eagerly conceded a cocaine exception to the traditional discretion of the individual druggist. Drug manufacturers made similar efforts, and a number of companies voluntarily discontinued the manufacture of coca and cocaine products. The support of cocaine control, in both instances, was one way to attack the "unprofessional" elements of medicine and pharmacy. For doctors and druggists, cocaine control merged with a broader effort to discipline the profession. For drug makers, cocaine control became a tool with which to attack the patent medicine industry and privilege the status of ethical and scientific drug manufacturers.[10]

Finally, the dual impulse explains some of the stranger results of early cocaine control. The most notable of these was the destruction of a formerly substantial market in low-potency coca preparations. Reformers were not blind to the differences among products; they understood that long-term use of most catarrh cures, for example, presented greater risks than most coca wines or voice tablets. The medical era actually saw fairly sharp distinctions drawn between the pharmacology of coca and that of cocaine, and yet the coca products were the target of relentless criticism because they fell on the wrong side of the industry. Here, the failure to exercise objective judgment reflected neither the ignorance of the age nor the unthinking zeal of the social reformer, but rather cold, political calculations that were built into the very foundation of modern drug control.

The Creation of the Cocaine Fiend

It is doubtful that the cocaine question could have achieved the prominence that it did merely on the strength of professional conflicts in medicine and pharmacy. The figure that animated reform was the cocaine fiend — the archetype of the modern drug taker and the object of control. The creation of the cocaine fiend, made up of equal parts of fear and fantasy, reveals the strengths of the constructionist perspective.

The fiend of popular imagination came from small truths magnified through lenses of fear, racism, and class prejudice. The control coalition clearly feared the results of the widespread use of cocaine among specific groups and did much to disseminate information that reinforced these negative images. The medical community was hardly immune; the iatrogenically addicted cocaine habitué during the medical era might have been regarded as having little or no control over his or her drug use, whereas the cocaine fiend appeared merely self-indulgent.

Yet the construction of the cocaine fiend required no formal controls. A legal supply of cocaine, even under medical authority, did not mean that cocaine taking was free of social or moral stigma. Indeed, one of the most remarkable aspects of the de-legitimation of cocaine taking was the emergence of an underground cocaine market before prohibition. In fact, this underground market is one of the surest signs that anticocaine sentiment had a practical impact on the lives of buyers and sellers. The informal limits on cocaine selling, together with the imposition of formal regulatory requirements, created an environment in which the legal market was unwilling or unable to meet the demands of popular use. By 1900, fifteen years before the Harrison Act and twenty-two years before the Jones-Miller Act, many users had clearly been forced to purchase cocaine from retailers who specialized in the cocaine trade to meet this unsatisfied demand. The regulated drug market therefore began to develop a number of features more commonly associated with the postprohibition black market: cocaine selling became increasingly geographically concentrated, usually coexisting with other underground trades in urban areas; the bulk of retail sales shifted from pharmacists to drug peddlers; and the product available to consumers declined in quality and purity. Moreover, the retail price of cocaine began to separate from the legal price, as the specialized cocaine sellers began to exact a premium for their willingness to cross lines of legitimate trade. That so many consumers were willing to pay that price is testimony to their unequal access to legal supplies.

The construction of the cocaine fiend was also a two-way process in which the drug takers themselves played an important role. The subjects of modern reform were themselves active agents in the creation of a drug culture and a shadow market.[11] The "cocaine flats" and "snow pads" of the underground market were more than mere refuges from the scorn of legitimate society or the prying eyes of the police. In important ways, buyers and sellers of cocaine developed their own networks of association which were as much a conscious statement of difference as they were an adaptation to the anticocaine movement. Creating a descriptive language of its own, with terms such as *Brighteye* used to describe cocaine, the new drug underground articulated the distance between themselves and the medical/social boundaries of legitimate cocaine use.

A narrow definition of drug history, with the conventional periodization of *before* and *after* prohibition, exaggerates the historical significance of the legal status of cocaine. Both critics and supporters of prohibitionist policies have taken this approach, and both equate much too facilely the acceptability and accessibility of a drug with its legal status. This easy equation was not true in the past, nor is it true today.

Modern drug control must be understood as the continuation of a process that began much earlier. That process had four basic elements, none of which is intelligible without reference to the others. First is the ongoing observation and measurement of drug effects. This was largely a medical/scientific function, although it has evolved during the twentieth century into a more specialized function of drug treatment providers and public health organizations. The critical information, for control purposes, involved the physical and mental harms caused by particular substances. In the case of cocaine, this information was then used to begin to define the boundaries of legitimate use.

Second is the regulation of drug manufacture, sale, and distribution. Originally the domain of individual manufacturers and retailers, this function was gradually taken over and formalized by the state (with the acquiescence of the drug business). This area of control focuses on the exchanges between buyer and seller; both must meet certain standards for a transaction to be appropriate.

Third, drug users themselves become the object of observation and study. Since the earliest years of the cocaine experience, the central preoccupation has been the attempt to define the nature and degree of difference between drug takers and "normal" people. Although the most obvious arena for this is medical and social scientific research, the process of definition happens at all levels of society.

Finally, drug takers themselves are engaged in an ongoing process of self-definition. The creation of a shadow market in cocaine would not have been necessary without the impact of formal and informal controls, but the character of that shadow market is understandable only through the daily actions of buyers and sellers. The four elements are not easily disentangled, and none is wholly dependent on the current state of legislation. Together, they have produced a century of drug wars that, for better or worse, mirror the time and place in which they are fought.

NOTES

Introduction

1. Papers delivered at the Hoover Conference on U.S. Drug Policy at Stanford University reveal the extent of interest in introducing some historical dimension to policy analysis. No less than half of the papers employed some form of historical analogy, usually to alcohol prohibition, whereas Ethan Nadelmann observed that "virtually nothing has been written" about the important question of cocaine use before controls on distribution. See Melvyn B. Krauss and Edward P. Lazear, eds., *Searching for Alternatives: Drug-Control Policy in the United States* (Stanford: Hoover Institution Press, 1991).

2. Representative examples of these early historical treatments include Richard Ashley, *Cocaine: Its History, Uses, and Effects* (New York: Warner Books, 1976) and Joel L. Phillips and Ronald W. Wynne, *Cocaine: The Mystique and the Reality* (New York: Avon Books, 1980).

3. For opiates, see David T. Courtwright, *Dark Paradise: Opiate Addiction in America before 1940* (Cambridge: Harvard University Press, 1982). For alcohol, see W. J. Rorabaugh, *The Alcoholic Republic* (New York: Oxford University Press, 1979).

4. A growing literature deals with constructionist aspects of drugs and addiction, including Stanton Peele, *Diseasing of America: Addiction Treatment Out of Control* (Lexington, Mass.: Lexington Books, 1989); Craig Reinarman and Harry G. Levine, "The Crack Attack: Politics and Media in America's Latest Drug Scare," in *Images of Issues: Typifying Contemporary Social Problems*, ed. Joel Best (New York: Aldine de Gruyter, 1989); and Norman Zinberg, *Drug, Set, and Setting: The Basis for Controlled Intoxicant Use* (New Haven: Yale University Press, 1984).

5. Joseph R. Gusfield, *Symbolic Crusade: Status Politics and the American Temperance Movement* (Urbana: University of Illinois Press, 1963); Marek Kohn, *Dope Girls: The Birth of the British Drug Underground* (London: Lawrence & Wishart, 1992).

6. Charles W. Collins and John Day, "Nightmare of Cocaine," *Everyday Life* (September 1909): 4–5.

7. Thomas G. Simonton, "The Increase of the Use of Cocaine among the Laity of Pittsburgh," *Philadelphia Medical Journal* 11 (March 28, 1903): 556; Charles Merriam Papers, vol. 88, folders 1, 6, and 7, University of Chicago special collections, Joseph Regenstein Library, Chicago, Ill.

8. Vincenzo Ruggerio and Nigel South, *Eurodrugs: Drug Use, Markets, and Trafficking in Europe* (London: UCL Press, 1995); Patricia Adler, *Wheeling and Dealing: An Ethnography of an Upper-Level Drug Dealing and Smuggling Community* (New York: Columbia University Press, 1985); Terry Williams, *The Cocaine Kids: The Inside Story of a Teenage Drug Ring* (Reading, Mass.: Addison-Wesley, 1989); Mark H. Haller, "Illegal Enterprise: Historical Perspectives and Public Policy," in *History and Crime: Implications for Criminal Jus-*

tice Policy, ed. James A. Inciardi and Charles E. Faupel (Beverly Hills, Calif.: Sage Publications, 1980).

9. Ethan A. Nadelmann, "Should We Legalize Drugs? History Answers," *American Heritage* (February/March 1993): 42–48.

10. Charles A. Bunting, *Hope for the Victims of Alcohol, Opium, Morphine, Cocaine, and Other Vices* (New York, 1888), 71.

One   A Miracle of Modern Science

1. Robert Byck, "Cocaine Use and Research: Three Histories," in *Cocaine: Clinical and Biobehavioral Aspects,* ed. Seymour Fischer, Allen Raskin, and E. H. Uhlenhuth (New York: Oxford University Press, 1987), 3–18. Byck's essay points out that medical knowledge of cocaine pharmacology was fairly advanced by the early twentieth century.

2. The testimony is that of a Swiss naturalist, Von Schuldi, who visited South America in 1838. His report is cited in W. Golden Mortimer, *Peru: History of Coca, "The Divine Plant" of the Incas* (New York, 1901), 171–72. Mortimer, an advocate of the therapeutic use of coca (which he carefully distinguished from the use of cocaine), was a distinguished surgeon and member of the New York Academy of Medicine. His monograph is an enormous work, covering nearly every aspect of the history and therapeutic use of coca.

3. Mortimer, *Peru: History of Coca,* 23.

4. John Uri Lloyd, *Origin and History of All the Pharmacopeial Vegetable Drugs* (Cincinnati, 1929), 92. Lloyd was a prominent eclectic physician and founder of the Lloyd Brothers pharmaceutical company. Lloyd, like other advocates of botanical medicine, placed great reliance on preparations of plant-based drugs — coca rather than cocaine, for example. Lloyd was also an outspoken critic of the devaluation of empirical observation in medicine. The works of the Lloyd brothers and their marvelous collection of pharmaceutical literature are in the Lloyd Library in Cincinnati.

5. Mortimer, *Peru: History of Coca,* appendix.

6. The coca experience presents a notable contrast to that of tobacco. Unlike coca, tobacco survived the long voyages to Europe in excellent condition, ready for consumption and with its stimulant properties intact.

7. William S. Searle, *A New Form of Nervous Disease (Together with an Essay on Erythroxylon Coca)* (New York, 1881), 107–11.

8. John Harley Warner, *The Therapeutic Perspective: Medical Practice, Knowledge, and Identity in America, 1820–1885* (Cambridge: Harvard University Press, 1986), 7.

9. E. R. Palmer, *Louisville Medical News* (1880); reprint, *The Pharmacology of the Newer Materia Medica,* 394–95.

10. G. F. Dowdeswell, "The Coca Leaf, Observations on the Properties and Action of the Leaf of the Coca Plant (Erythroxylon Coca), Made in the Physiological Laboratory of University College," *Lancet* (1876): 631, 664.

11. Searle, *A New Form of Nervous Disease,* 117–18.

12. Lloyd, *Origin and History,* 99–100.

13. Edward R. Squibb, "Report on the Drug Market," *Proceedings of the American Pharmaceutical Association* 11 (1863): 175–95; reprint, *The Collected Papers of Edward Robinson Squibb, M.D., 1819–1900,* vol. 1, ed. Klaus Florey (Squibb Corporation, 1988), 301–21.

14. E. R. Squibb, "Erythroxylon Coca," *Pharmaceutical Journal and Transactions* 15 (Au-

gust 23, 1884): 145–47, in *Collected Papers of Edward Robinson Squibb*, 1217–19. It should be noted that the figure of 40 million pounds of coca represents total consumption, nearly all consumed in the producing countries of Peru, Bolivia, and Ecuador.

15. Roberts Bartholow described the rapid response to Koller's new application of cocaine: "As the possibilities of the future utility of cocaine as a local anesthetic were then recognized, it created a profound impression, and in an incredibly short time this remarkable discovery became the common interest and the common possession. Everywhere cocaine was investigated by physiological and clinical methods, and the results confirmed the statements of Koller." Roberts Bartholow, *A Practical Treatise on Materia Medica and Therapeutics*, 10th ed. (New York, 1900), 558.

16. William Oliver Moore, "The Physiological and Therapeutical Effects of the Coca-Leaf and Its Alkaloid," *New York Medical Journal* 41 (January 3, 1885): 19–23.

17. *Index-Catalogue of the Library of the Surgeon-General's Office, United States Army*, 2d series, 3 (Washington, D.C.: GPO, 1898), 701–4.

18. C. H. Castle, "Observations upon the Hydro-Chlorate of Cocaine, with Some Special Studies upon Its Effects on Accommodation," *Medical News* 45 (December 6, 1884): 622; Francke H. Bosworth, "A New Therapeutic Use for Cocaine," *Medical Record* 26 (November 15, 1884): 533–34.

19. J. M. DaCosta, "Some Observations on the Use of the Hydrochloride of Cocaine, Especially Its Hypodermic Use," *Medical News* 45 (December 13, 1884): 651–54.

20. Bartholow, *A Practical Treatise*, 558; J. H. Warner writes, "Bartholow was exemplary of those American physicians who were most optimistic about the promise of experimental laboratory science to transform therapeutics and rouse the profession from its gloom. Therapeutics 'is an experimental science,' he claimed, and some of its facts 'are capable of the same kind of experimental proof as are the facts of the biological sciences.' The empiricism of the Paris clinical school had proved inadequate in effecting positive progress and giving the practitioner assured therapeutic confidence at the bedside, physicians like Bartholow believed." Warner, *Therapeutic Perspective*, 257.

21. "Cocaine Hydrochloride, the New Local Anesthetic," *Maryland Medical Journal* (1884): 513.

22. Francke H. Bosworth, "An Additional Note on the Therapeutic Action of Cocaine," *New York Medical Journal* 43 (March 20, 1886): 323. See also E. W. Holmes, "Erythroxylon Coca and Its Alkaloid Cocaine," *Therapeutic Gazette* (1886): 526.

23. E. R. Squibb, "Cocaine," *Pharmaceutical Journal and Transactions* 15 (December 15, 1884): 465; reprint, *Collected Papers*, 1236. The switch to positive reviews of cocaine caused some comment. John Uri Lloyd, although critical of Squibb's earlier condemnation of the drug, praised him for recognizing the new information and admitting its importance. The editor of the *Medical Register* was not nearly as charitable, however. Referring to Squibb's role in medicine as that of an "ignoramus and an obstructionist," the journal called his actions with regard to cocaine "both ignorant and inconsistent" and accused him of manipulating the drug market through the pages of his scientific journal. "The Squibb Issue," *Medical Register* (1887): 517–18; reprint, *Collected Papers*, 1286–87.

24. See, for example, the comments of North Carolina laryngologist C. P. Ambler, "Cocaine: Its Uses and Abuses," *Cleveland Medical Gazette* 10 (1894–95): 54–62.

25. Le Roy Pope Walker, "A Few Clinical Facts Regarding Cocaine Hydrochloride, The New Anesthetic," *New York Medical Journal* 40 (October 25, 1884): 459–60. In the same

report, Walker reported on thirteen other patients, and in nearly each case he noted the lack of "resistance" offered by the patient. See M. D. Hoge, "Therapeutics of Cocaine, with Some Personal Experimental Observations," *Virginia Medical Monthly* 13 (1886–87): 301–11.

26. See Martin S. Pernick, *A Calculus of Suffering: Pain, Professionalism and Anesthesia in Nineteenth-Century America* (New York: Columbia University Press, 1985), 211. The introduction of cocaine was one of several changes in the late nineteenth century which increasingly promoted surgical specialization. For the development of late-nineteenth-century surgical practice, I have found the following useful: William G. Rothstein, *American Physicians in the Nineteenth Century* (Baltimore: Johns Hopkins University Press, 1972), especially chap. 13, "The Beginnings of Scientific Medicine: Surgery"; and Gert H. Brieger, "Surgery," in *The Education of American Physicians: Historical Essays,* ed. Ronald L. Numbers (Berkeley, Calif: University of California Press, 1980).

27. Pernick, *A Calculus of Suffering,* 237.

28. T. R. Pooley, "Some Observations in the Use of the Hydrochloride of Cocaine," *New England Medicine Monthly* 4 (1884–85): 264–70.

29. Moore, "The Physiological and Therapeutical Effects of Coca-Leaf and Its Alkaloid," 22.

30. William Chapman Jarvis, "Cocaine in Nasal Surgery," *Medical Record* (December 13, 1884); reprint, *The Pharmacology of the Newer Materia Medica* (Detroit: George S. Davis, 1892), 479–80.

31. On the relationship between neurology and the emerging field of psychology, see Stephen Young Wilkerson, "Mind over Body: James Jackson Putnam and the Impact of Neurology on Psychotherapy in Late Nineteenth-Century America" (Ph.D. diss., Duke University, 1978); Gerald Grob, *Mental Illness and American Society, 1875–1940* (Princeton: Princeton University Press, 1983), and Nathan G. Hale Jr., *Freud and the Americans: The Beginnings of Psychoanalysis in the United States, 1876–1917* (New York: Oxford University Press, 1971). See also Bonnie Ellen Blustein, "A New York Medical Man: William Alexander Hammond, M.D. (1828–1900), Neurologist" (Ph.D. diss., University of Pennsylvania, 1979).

32. George M. Beard, *American Nervousness: Its Causes and Consequences* (New York, 1881), title page. *American Nervousness* was the follow-up work to the groundbreaking work by Beard, *A Practical Treatise on Nervous Exhaustion (Neurasthenia): Its Symptoms, Nature, Sequences, Treatment* (New York, 1880). There are numerous historical works on neurasthenia, including Francis G. Gosling, "American Nervousness: A Study in Medicine and Social Values in the Gilded Age, 1870–1900" (Ph.D. diss., University of Oklahoma, 1976); and Tom Lutz, *American Nervousness, 1903* (Ithaca: Cornell University Press, 1991).

33. Searle, *A New Form of Nervous Disease,* 134–35.

34. Beard, *A Practical Treatise on Nervous Exhaustion,* 151–52; D. R. Brower, "The Effects of Cocaine on the Central Nervous System," *Medical Age* 4 (1886): 27–32. Beard's commentary illustrates further the skepticism that many held for coca before 1884.

35. Horatio C. Wood, *Therapeutics: Its Principles and Practice,* 8th ed. (Philadelphia, 1891), 246.

36. Sigmund Freud, *Uber Coca* (July 1884); reprint, *Cocaine Papers by Sigmund Freud,* ed. Robert Byck (New York: Stonehill, 1975). Byck has assembled the best collection of primary documents detailing the therapeutic use of cocaine. Although Freud's first work was

published in German in July 1884, the first appearance in the American literature of this work was in the November 1886 issue of the *St. Louis Medical Journal*. Clearly, Freud deserves some credit for being among the first to apply cocaine as a stimulant and in the treatment of opiate addiction. As Byck makes clear, however, Freud's work was clearly derivative of the earlier American work with coca. Moreover, after Koller's announcement in late 1884, many American physicians carried on similar work without any knowledge of Freud's studies. Freud's studies are tremendously valuable — they remain today some of the most complete studies of cocaine action — but they did not have the influence on medical practice which Koller's breakthrough did.

37. Francis E. Stewart, "Coca Leaf Cigars and Cigarettes," *Philadelphia Medical Times* 15 (September 19, 1885): 933–35.

38. Walter Woodman, "Cocaine For Sleeplessness," *Boston Medical and Surgical Journal* 112 (1885): 287.

39. The case originally appeared in the *Ohio Medical Journal*, was reprinted by the *Medical Record* of New York, and used by D. R. Brower in a report to the Chicago Medical Society.

40. Brower, "The Effects of Cocaine," 27; the most frequently cited example of cocaine as a mental stimulant is Arthur Conan Doyle's fictional cocaine user, Sherlock Holmes. As often as the detective's cocaine use is cited, it is rarely described in its therapeutic context. Conan Doyle, a physician, included cocaine in his stories written during the height of the medical use of cocaine during the 1880s. At the time, many physicians and other "brain workers" (undoubtedly some of his acquaintance) were using cocaine as a mental stimulant. The description of the effect of cocaine by Holmes (perhaps the most famous fictional brain worker) in *The Sign of Four* (1888) is one of the best examples of medical thought on the action of cocaine.

41. Stewart, "Coca Leaf Cigars and Cigarettes."

42. James W. Hole, *Therapeutic Gazette* (1880) in *The Pharmacology of the Newer Materia Medica*, ed. George S. Davis (Detroit, 1892), 393–94.

43. J. Chalmers DaCosta, "Four Cases of Cocaine Delirium," *Philadelphia Neurological Society* (1889): 193; W. A. Hammond, "Cocaine and the So-Called Cocaine Habit," *New York Medical Journal* 44 (1886): 637–39; Brower, "The Effects of Cocaine," 28.

44. The case of Grant's illness is an interesting one; although some coca wine was given as a tonic and support, the treatment of his illness was more notable for the use of cocaine (in solution) as a topical anesthetic. As Grant labored to complete his memoirs in early 1885, Douglas continued to apply cocaine to alleviate some of his patient's pain. Grant occasionally refused the topical applications of cocaine, however, saying that the drug impaired his already limited ability to speak. Thomas M. Pitkin, *The Captain Departs: Ulysses S. Grant's Last Campaign* (Carbondale, Ill.: Southern Illinois University Press, 1973), 31, 69, 79.

45. Lewis H. Adler Jr., "The Status of the Uses of Cocaine in General Medicine," *International Medical Magazine* 2 (1893–94): 246–61, 305–13.

46. David T. Courtwright, *Dark Paradise: Opiate Addiction in America before 1940* (Cambridge: Harvard University Press, 1982). See also idem, "The Hidden Epidemic: Opiate Addiction and Cocaine Use in the South, 1860–1920," *Journal of Southern History* 49 (February 1983): 57–72.

47. Courtwright, *Dark Paradise*, especially chap. 2, "Addiction to Opium and Mor-

phine"; the most comprehensive examination of changing therapeutic dosages and forms of opiates is in Warner, *The Therapeutic Perspective,* chap. 4, "Therapeutic Change."

48. G. H. Gray, "Coca in the Opium Habit," *Therapeutic Gazette* 2 (1881): 231–32; H. F. Stimmell, "Coca in the Opium and Alcohol Habits," *Therapeutic Gazette* 2 (1881).

49. W. H. Bentley, "Erythroxylon Coca in the Opium and Alcohol Habits," *New Orleans Medical and Surgical Journal* 8 (November 1880): 471–72; Gray, "Coca in the Opium Habit."

50. Freud, *Uber Coca,* 69–72.

51. Beard, *American Nervousness.* Neurologists and inebriety specialists often classified alcohol inebriety in the same manner. In his study on coca Mortimer claimed that it could be useful in this kind of inebriety, as "drunkenness may simply be a manifestation of a diseased nervous system."

52. J. T. Whittaker, "Cocaine in the Treatment of the Opium Habit," *Medical News* 47 (August 8, 1885): 144–49.

53. Bosworth, "A New Therapeutic Use for Cocaine."

54. Seth S. Bishop, *Cocaine in Hay Fever* (Chicago: American Medical Association, 1886).

55. Bartholow, *A Practical Treatise,* 561.

56. Bishop, *Cocaine in Hay Fever,* 9.

57. Mortimer, *Peru: History of Coca,* 501–7.

58. Hoge, "Therapeutics of Cocaine," 305.

59. Brower, "The Effects of Cocaine," 31.

60. Lester Grinspoon and James B. Bakalar, *Cocaine: A Drug and Its Social Evolution* (New York: Basic Books, 1976), 23–24.

61. Adler, "The Status of the Uses of Cocaine in General Medicine."

Two   Debating the Dangers of Cocaine

1. David Musto suggests that the medical community was "enthusiastic and sincerely uncritical" in its response to cocaine. He then describes a "second stage" during which physicians gradually became aware of the "casualties" of cocaine use, and the drug fell into disfavor. David F. Musto, "Lessons of the First Cocaine Epidemic," the *Wall Street Journal* (June 11, 1986): 31. A recent work asserts that cocaine fell rapidly from "wonder drug" to unwanted drug and goes so far as to suggest that because physicians recognized the undesirability of cocaine use, it was "unfortunate" that the story of cocaine was "not simply a tale of scientists and medical practitioners." John C. Flynn, *Cocaine: An In-Depth Look at the Facts, Science, History and Future of the World's Most Addictive Drug* (New York: Birch Lane Press, 1991), 22.

2. I have chosen in this chapter to refer to *cocaine habit* and *habitué.* In describing the phenomenon in the 1880s and 1890s, *cocaine habit* was the preferred language, and in most instances, I have retained that term. I do so because the term *addict* is problematic, given the current disputes over the nature of cocaine use and misuse. In some instances, when paraphrasing historical speakers, I have retained the term *addict,* but I avoid entirely currently popular terms such as *dependence* or *abuse.*

3. The reports are in J. B. Mattison, "Cocaine Dosage and Cocaine Addiction," *Peoria Medical Monthly* 7 (1886–87): 532–42, 571–81; and idem, "Cocaine Toxemia," *Quarterly*

Journal of Inebriety 10 (1888): 57–67. Mattison had, a decade earlier, been a leading critic of the overuse of chloral hydrate in the medical profession. The following is a summary of the origins of Mattison's sixty-eight cases: local anesthetic (forty cases); local anesthetic, dentistry (ten cases); general analgesia (five cases); tonic and stimulant (four cases); hay fever (three cases); self-experimentation (two cases); nausea (one case); accidental (one case); and unknown (two cases).

4. In reporting dosages, it should be noted that nearly all physicians in the United States measured amounts in grains. Today, most similar measurements would either be in milligrams or grams. Therefore, in some instances both gram measurements and grain measurements are given.

5. Few, if any, reliable cases of deaths from social/recreational cocaine were ever reported. Richard Ashley noted the same phenomenon in his work *Cocaine: Its History, Uses, and Effects* (New York: Warner Books, 1976) and suggested that this might serve to question the reliability of the reported cases of deaths (he noted thirteen by 1891). In fact, it seems likely that the reporting of the deaths was accurate. Social users of cocaine may adjust their dosage to safer levels, often increasing dosages over time. In its early surgical uses, large amounts of cocaine were injected, and if a patient were particularly sensitive to the drug little could be done (as with one of five fatalities reported by Mattison: a twenty-three-year-old woman was injected with nearly 2 grams of cocaine before removal of a lesion). One field with a large share of the reported deaths from toxic reactions was in operations on the urethra. The effects of cocaine promised surgeons and others greater ease in examining the urethra as well. For several reasons, large amounts of cocaine were often injected to produce anesthesia. A detailed description of a fatal reaction is given in J. Henry C. Simes, "The Injection of a Solution of Cocaine into the Urethra followed by Death," *Medical News* 53 (July 21, 1888): 70–71. In early 1887, several medical journals reported a tragic case of cocaine poisoning from St. Petersburg. A young Russian surgeon named Kolomnin injected 24 grains of cocaine (1.55 grams) into a patient before attempting to remove a rectal ulcer. As the *Boston Medical and Surgical Journal* reported, "twenty or thirty minutes afterward, symptoms of poisoning declared themselves, syncope and complete collapse set in, and in spite of stimulants, injections of ether, faradization, artificial respiration, etc., the patient died." Compounding the tragedy, the young surgeon committed suicide after the death.

6. E. W. Holmes, "Erythroxylon Coca and Its Alkaloid Cocaine," *Therapeutic Gazette* (1886): 526–31.

7. S. Mitchell, "Coffee in Cocaine-Poisoning," *Medical Record* 37 (May 31, 1890): 616.

8. Stickler's cases are reported in the following: J. W. Stickler, "Peculiar Effect of Cocaine," *Medical Record* 31 (March 19, 1887): 325; idem, "Another Peculiar Effect of Cocaine," *Medical Record* 37 (1890): 238–39; idem, "The Awakening Effect of Cocaine," *Medical Record* 45 (January 13, 1894): 59.

9. G. E. Pettey, "Cocaine as a Respiratory Stimulant," *Southern Medical Journal* 7 (1914): 273–74.

10. M. D. Hoge, "Therapeutics of Cocaine, with Some Personal Experimental Observations," *Virginia Medical Monthly* 13 (August 1886): 301–11.

11. D. S. Booth, "Cocaine Poisoning," *Medical Standard* 4 (1888): 100.

12. Mattison, "Cocaine Dosage and Cocaine Addiction," 572–73.

13. A. P. Cornell, "Is Cocaine Aphrodisiac?" *Medical Brief* 19 (1891): 152. Cornell noted

that the girl's father was standing nearby "but fortunately did not hear her words, or understand her actions."

14. J. Chalmers DaCosta, "Four Cases of Cocaine Delirium," *Philadelphia Neurological Society* (1889): 188–94.

15. Ibid., 192–94.

16. D. R. Brower, "The Effects of Cocaine on the Central Nervous System," *Medical Age* 4 (1886): 27–32.

17. Robert Cohn, "On a Case of Cocaine Poisoning," *Occidental Medical Times* 17 (1903): 241–42. This point of view appears in some leading medical texts as well, including Roberts Bartholow, *A Practical Treatise on Materia Medica and Therapeutics,* 10th ed. (New York, 1900), 559.

18. Isidor Gluck, "The Prevention of the Toxic Effect of Cocaine," *Medical Record* 37 (June 21, 1890): 707.

19. W. Sheppegrell, "The Abuse and Dangers of Cocain," *Medical News* 73 (October 1, 1898): 417–22.

20. Lewis H. Adler Jr., "The Status of the Uses of Cocaine in General Medicine," *International Medical Magazine* 2 (1893–94): 246–61, 305–13.

21. Lewis H. Adler, "The Status of the Hydrochloride of Cocaine in Minor Surgery, as Based upon the Experiences of Philadelphia Physicians," *Therapeutic Gazette* 7 (1891): 518–33. Adler's results are echoed in other surgical reports, such as William H. Dukeman, "Cocaine in Urethral Surgery," *New York Medical Journal* 62 (September 21, 1895): 369.

22. Charles H. Chetwood, "The Toxic Effect of Cocaine Hydrochloride, with Report of a Case," *Medical Record* 36 (August 10, 1889): 144–45.

23. Mattison, "Cocaine Dosage and Cocaine Addiction," 532.

24. J. T. Whittaker, "Cocaine in the Treatment of the Opium Habit," *Medical News* 47 (August 8, 1885): 144–49.

25. William A. Hammond, "Cocaine and the So-called Cocaine Habit," *New York Medical Journal* 44 (1886): 637–39.

26. David Musto concludes, for example, that there was "little desire to listen to killjoys" among those physicians who used cocaine. Musto, "Lessons of the First Cocaine Epidemic." The contrary interpretation has been that these voices represented the truth about cocaine, which was (and continues to be) stifled by irrational fears. Richard Ashley described the fears of early medical critics as "misplaced, to say the least." Ashley and others make the observation that medical claims of cocaine's dangers were likely based on economic self-interest; when patent medicine interests took over the sale of cocaine, physicians no longer felt constrained to support its use. Ashley, *Cocaine,* 75.

27. Adler, "The Status of the Uses of Cocaine in General Medicine," 246–61, 305–13.

28. It should also be noted that no cases of the coca habit or cocaine habit through oral dosage were noted in the medical literature. Although it was later suggested that coca, like cocaine, had addictive potential, this is not confirmed by the historical data.

29. Adler, "The Status of the Uses of Cocaine in General Medicine," 246–61, 305–13.

30. Ibid., 255.

31. Ibid., 260.

32. Some cocaine users found that its effects also balanced the effects of alcohol or of a hangover. The *Medical Record* published an account of a Marine private who went on an alcohol- and cocaine-using binge and afterwards administered hypodermically "a dose to

sober up." J. S. Spear, "A Case of Cocaine Poisoning Simulating Opium Poisoning," *Medical Record* 28 (November 14, 1885): 536.

33. Heine Marks, "The General Treatment of Habitual and Periodical Alcoholic, Morphine, and Cocaine Inebriates," *Quarterly Journal of Inebriety* 18 (1896): 148.

34. These figures reflect average daily use of cocaine as given in twenty-eight case histories.

35. Judson B. Andrews, "Report of Two Cases of Morphia and Cocaine Habit," *Transactions of the New York Medical Association* 3 (1886): 68–77.

36. H. G. Brainerd, "Cocaine Addiction," *Transactions of the Medical Society of the State of California* (1891): 200.

37. Robert W. Haynes, "The Dangers of Cocain," *Medical News* 65 (1894): 14.

38. T. D. Crothers, "Some Medico-Legal Questions Concerning Cocaine Inebriety," *Medicine* 2 (1896): 298.

39. J. W. Springthorpe, "The Confessions of a Cocainist," *Quarterly Journal of Inebriety* 19 (1897): 55, 59.

40. Courtwright, *Dark Paradise: Opiate Addiction in America before 1940* (Cambridge: Harvard University Press, 1982). For a contemporary version, see Joseph B. Treaster, "Executive's Secret Struggle with Heroin's Powerful Grip," *New York Times* (July 22, 1992).

41. This conclusion is confirmed in a variety of sources. This is not to suggest that some users did not experience serious personal and career disruptions. Nor should this suggest that many addicts were not anxious to discontinue their use of opium and morphine. The popularity of various addiction cures, including cocaine, attests to their desire to break the habit.

42. Brainerd, "Cocaine Addiction," 200.

43. C. C. Stockard, "Some Cases of Drug Habit," *Atlanta Medical and Surgical Journal* 15 (1898–99): 83.

44. Charles A. Bunting, *Hope for the Victims of Alcohol, Opium, Morphine, Cocaine, and Other Vices* (New York, 1888), 71.

45. Hobart Amory Hare, *A Text-Book of Practical Therapeutics* (Philadelphia, 1895), 159.

46. Springthorpe, "The Confessions of a Cocainist," 58.

47. Andrews, "Report of Two Cases of Morphia and Cocaine Habit," 68–77.

48. Mattison, "Cocaine Dosage and Cocaine Addiction," 577–80.

49. Francke H. Bosworth, "An Additional Note on the Therapeutic Action of Cocaine," *New York Medical Journal* 43 (March 20, 1886): 323.

50. Seth S. Bishop, *Cocaine in Hay Fever* (Chicago: American Medical Association, 1886), 8–10.

51. Brower, "The Effects of Cocaine," 28.

52. Mattison, "Cocaine Dosage and Cocaine Addiction," 581.

53. Stockard, "Some Cases of Drug Habit," 80–81.

54. Adler, "The Status of the Uses of Cocaine in General Medicine," 259.

55. Marks, "The General Treatment," 153–54.

56. In his last paper published on the subject of cocaine, Freud responded to his critics by citing the work of Hammond. Published in America as "Remarks on the Craving for and Fear of Cocaine," Freud wrote "Dr. Hammond placed the habituation to cocaine on a par with that of coffee or tea, an entirely different sort of habit from morphia addiction. He did not believe that there is a single verified case of cocaine addiction on record (except

among morphine addicts), that is to say, of the sort in which the patient would be incapable of discontinuing use of the drug at will." Freud's work is reprinted in Byck, *Cocaine Papers by Sigmund Freud* (New York: Stonehill, 1975).

57. Brainerd, "Cocaine Addiction," 200.

58. Adler, "The Status of the Uses of Cocaine in General Medicine," 250.

59. Courtwright, *Dark Paradise.*

60. T. D. Crothers, "Cocaine-Inebriety," *Quarterly Journal of Inebriety* 20 (1898): 370.

61. E. W. Holmes, "Erythroxylon Coca and Its Alkaloid Cocaine," *Therapeutic Gazette* (1886): 531. As a warning to fellow physicians, Frank Ring published in 1887 an article entitled "Cocaine and Its Fascinations, from a Personal Experience," *Medical Record* 32 (September 3, 1887): 274. Ring concluded that this experience profoundly affected his perspective on using cocaine in his practice: "I would not be willing to take the responsibility of a like continuance with any patient; neither would I put it in the hands of one to be used at his discretion. Several times have I been asked, after spraying the nose, what that medicine was which produced such a marked relief in breathing. The answer is always: a solution of the erythroxylon plant. The words coca and cocaine are not in my vocabulary when addressing patients." Interestingly, his experience did not discourage his use altogether.

62. Bunting, *Hope for the Victims,* 71.

63. This explanation should be qualified by noting that even in the twentieth century, with more standardized testing and evaluation processes for new drugs, physicians continue to have one of the highest rates of addiction. This phenomenon suggests that abuse is also partially a result of exposure.

64. Haynes, "The Dangers of Cocain," 14.

65. The full story of Halsted's struggle with cocaine was not revealed until 1969, when a private history of Johns Hopkins Hospital by William Osler was first read. In his account, Osler revealed Halsted's replacement of cocaine with morphine.

66. Crothers, "Cocaine-Inebriety," 369–74.

67. Marks, "The General Treatment," 159.

68. Arnold Jaffe, "Addiction Reform in the Progressive Age" (Ph.D. diss., University of Kentucky, 1976; reprint, New York: Arno Press, 1981).

69. Brower, "The Effects of Cocaine," 29.

70. "Cocaine's Terrible Effect," *New York Times* (November 30, 1885).

71. Brower, "The Effects of Cocaine," 30.

72. Ibid., 29–31.

73. "The Cocaine Victim Improving," *New York Times* (December 9, 1885).

74. "Cocaine's Destructive Work," *New York Times* (January 25, 1887).

Three   Making Cocaine

1. "Anesthesia by the Local Use of Hydrochlorate of Cocaine," *American Druggist* 13 (November 1884): 210.

2. *Oil, Paint, and Drug Reporter* (hereafter *OPDR*) (November 19, 1884).

3. This chapter makes a careful distinction between chemical firms and pharmaceutical firms. Chemical companies specialized in the large-scale production of medicinal chemicals such as morphine, strychnine, and quinine. Pharmaceutical firms usually purchased

these products from chemical firms and used the drug in the preparation of dosage-level products or drug compounds.

4. C. N. Anderson, "Memoirs" (1936), Parke, Davis & Company Collection (hereafter PDC), Burton Historical Collection, Detroit Public Library; McKesson and Robbins' *Prices Current* and W. H. Schieffelin & Co. *General Prices Current*, American Institute for the History of Pharmacy collections.

5. Freud's early struggle with the expense of cocaine is recounted in Byck, *Cocaine Papers by Sigmund Freud* (New York: Stonehill, 1975).

6. "Gehe & Co. Semi-Annual Review of Drugs and Chemicals," *OPDR* (May 13, 1885).

7. John Uri Lloyd, *A Treatise on Coca (Erythroxylon Coca): "The Divine Plant of the Incas"* (Cincinnati, 1913), 15.

8. "Cocaine Hydrochlorate," *Pharmaceutical Record* (1884): 465.

9. William Oliver Moore, "The Physiological and Therapeutical Effects of the Coca-Leaf and Its Alkaloid," *New York Medical Journal* 41 (January 3, 1885): 19–23.

10. Henry Hurd Rusby, *Jungle Memories* (New York, 1933), 3.

11. For more on Rusby, see George A. Bender, "Henry Hurd Rusby: Scientific Explorer, Societal Crusader, Scholastic Innovator," *Pharmacy in History* 23 (1981): 70–85.

12. The response from Bolivian Consul-General Richard Gibbs included a wealth of detail on the Bolivian coca trade. His report was published in the *Pharmaceutical Record* that same year. Richard Gibbs, "On Coca," *Pharmaceutical Record* (March 1886): 14.

13. Much of the coca exports went to supply gauchos in Argentina and workers in the mines and nitrate fields of Chile.

14. The dual classification system had many confusing variants. As the *OPDR* suggested, "nothing is more striking than the uncertain manner in which the commercial varieties of the leaves are described." "The Cultivation of Coca," *OPDR* (February 13, 1887). The Hamburg drug market classified leaves as Huanuco, Truxillo, and Bolivian. The New York Quinine and Chemical Works described Huanuco, Truxillo, and Cuzco leaves. The German firm of Knoll & Company identified all four types of leaves: Huanuco, Truxillo, Bolivian, and Cuzco. See correspondence between Lyman Kebler and cocaine manufacturers during 1907 in the records of the Bureau of Chemistry (United States Department of Agriculture [hereafter USDA]), RG97, National Archives, Washington, D.C. (hereafter BC).

15. Advocates of the use of coca, such as W. Golden Mortimer and Angelo Mariani, concerned over the misuse of its alkaloid cocaine, used Rusby's reports to suggest that the physiological action of the coca leaf was different from that of cocaine. As Mortimer concluded, "Since 1885, most of the writings and the experiments of physiologists upon Coca seem to have been based upon the idea of a single active principle which should represent the potency of the leaf. . . this is a false supposition. The qualities of Coca are not fully represented by any one of its alkaloids thus far isolated." W. Golden Mortimer, *Peru: History of Coca, "The Divine Plant" of the Incas* (New York, 1901), 103.

16. What seems to have made one or another type of coca popular, though, had a great deal to do with cost. Truxillo leaves became popular with American cocaine manufacturers when the cost of Huanuco leaves increased substantially. As for the use of Truxillo leaves in coca products, manufacturers often paid little attention to the characteristics of the leaves when purchasing them through crude drug distributors or drug wholesalers. As the makers of Maltine Coca Wine suggested concerning coca leaves, "we buy anything we can get." Bureau of Chemistry hearing 64 "Maltine Coca Wine" (November 12, 1907): 14–15, BC.

17. "Coca Culture," *American Druggist* 20 (July 15, 1891): 214.

18. Edward R. Squibb, "Coca at the Source of Supply," *Pharmaceutical Journal and Transactions* (July 11, 1885): 46–49.

19. The weekly drug trade reports of the *OPDR* furnished most of the accounts of coca production and transportation.

20. "Coca: The Genus Erythroxylon," *American Druggist* 15 (April 1886): 86–88, 102, 115.

21. "The Decline in Cocaine," *OPDR* (April 29, 1895): 5.

22. Louis Lewin, *Phantastica: Narcotic and Stimulating Drugs, Their Use and Abuse* (1924; reprint, New York: E. P. Dutton, 1964), 77.

23. "Coca and Cocaine in Peru," *American Druggist* 30 (March 25, 1897): 174.

24. The effort to introduce coca cultivation was a quest that was ultimately frustrated by the lack of suitable climate conditions, which coca requires. In particular, no location possessed the combination of high altitude and a wet, temperate climate.

25. Merrill Collett, *The Cocaine Connection* (Headline Series, Foreign Policy Association, 1989), 13.

26. "Cocaine in Madras," *OPDR* (February 1, 1892): 45.

27. Lloyd, *A Treatise on Coca.*

28. "Coca: Its Properties and Principles," *National Druggist* (February 27, 1885): 113–15.

29. In fact, British India was one of the first areas, outside of the United States, to develop a serious problem with the overuse of cocaine. The first restrictions on the sale and use of cocaine were imposed in Bengal in 1902, about the same time as the first state regulations in the United States. The Bombay and Madras governments followed suit in 1903 and 1906, followed by all of British India in 1908. See, for example, *Chemist and Druggist* (February 17, 1906): 282, which notes that the Indian government banned the sale of cocaine from Calcutta by requiring dealers there to register with the government.

30. "How Drugs Are Imported," *American Druggist* 19 (July 1890): 126.

31. One issue about which historians have only recently begun to learn more is the development of coca production on the island of Formosa in the 1920s. This venture was led by the emerging Japanese chemical industry, but there is little evidence of how much cocaine ever resulted from its efforts. One suggestive note appears in a *Chicago Tribune* report of 1923, which claimed that three million forged Merck labels had been shipped from Germany to China, where they were put on bottles of Japanese cocaine. Because the smallest unit of manufacture distributed by chemical companies was 1/8 ounce, this represents at least 375,000 ounces of cocaine. In addition, director Hecht of Merck claimed that Japanese production was "probably more" than that of Germany in 1923. "Illicit Traffic in Drugs Runs Allied Cordon," *Chicago Sunday Tribune* (May 20, 1923): 7.

32. Coca seeds had been transported for planting in Java as far back as 1854, but the medical director of the government of the Dutch East Indies had declared their planting to be "dangerous for the colony." *Merck's Report* described the Javanese plantations in poetic fashion: "The light-green luxuriant foliage of coca bushes, that carpet the rolling hillsides for miles around, contrasting with the dark green foliage of the trees of adjoining rubber estates, while all is surrounded by dark depths of virgin forests, makes a landscape that is beautiful indeed." "A Coca Plantation in Java," *National Druggist* (April 1917): 135.

33. Rusby, *Jungle Memories,* 345.

34. "Cultivation of the Coca Plant in the United States," *National Druggist* (February 1885): 70.

35. Anderson, "Memoirs," PDC.

36. When Edmundo Morales interviewed a young Peruvian manufacturer of coca paste in the early 1980s, the man's eighty-year-old grandfather recalled that in his youth, he had met Germans arriving to set up cocaine factories. Morales notes parenthetically that the old man probably meant Anglos, but he may indeed have dealt with German manufacturers early in the century. Edmundo Morales, *Cocaine: White Gold Rush in Peru* (Tucson: University of Arizona Press, 1989), 75.

37. "Notes on Coca and Cocaine," *American Druggist* 44 (April 10, 1905): 201–2.

38. In most instances, the functions of coca harvesting and coca processing were also separated, although some large plantation owners expressed an interest in establishing crude cocaine manufactories of their own (I have not located any record of whether such facilities were ever established).

39. "The Manufacture of Cocaine in Peru," *American Druggist* 45 (October 17, 1904): 262.

40. Ibid.

41. "Illicit Traffic in Drugs Runs Allied Cordon," 7.

42. American manufacturers fought the 25 percent duty on crude cocaine for years, arguing that the duty imposed an unreasonable burden on potential manufacturers. The 25 percent duty originally applied to the finished product as well; imported cocaine hydrochloride was limited because of the added expense. Importers and German manufacturers successfully argued their case that imported cocaine hydrochloride should be subject to the duty of 50¢ per pound on medicinal preparations. Repeated challenges in the 1890s to the status of crude cocaine as a "manufactured article" rather than a "medicinal preparation" by Mallinckrodt Chemical Works and Lehn & Fink failed.

43. H. B. Rosengarten to USDA, Bureau of Chemistry, October 7, 1907, BC.

44. Almost as soon as manufacturers began offering cocaine in packages of variable amounts, a price scale replaced the initial standard per-grain cost. Thus, for example, the McKesson & Robbins wholesale catalog for 1887 offered the following: 5-grain vials for 10¢, 10-grain vials for 19¢, 15-grain vials for 28¢, 1/8-ounce vials for $1.00, and 1-ounce vials for $7.50. In this instance, McKesson & Robbins offered its customers per-grain price ranging between 2 and 1.7¢.

45. Editorial, *OPDR* (February 17, 1886): 5.

46. E. R. Squibb, "Hydrochlorate of Cocaine," *Pharmaceutical Record* (1884): 27.

47. Charles L. Huisking, *Herbs to Hormones: The Evolution of Drugs and Chemicals That Revolutionized Medicine* (Essex, Conn.: Pequot Press, 1968), 136.

48. Pharmaceutical manufacturers imported or produced their own botanical products and basic extracts or preparations of these botanicals. Pharmaceutical manufacturers did not require chemical companies to supply them with opium, for example, but they did require chemical companies to supply most of their morphine (and later, heroin).

49. Merck & Co. began its life primarily as an importer of goods manufactured in Germany by E. Merck. E. Merck & Company established manufacturing facilities in New Jersey in 1903, became officially incorporated in 1908, and broke from its German parent firm during World War I.

50. The leading cocaine manufacturer by all accounts was Germany; the United States, for a time, was the second largest producer of cocaine. Other European nations also had companies producing substantial amounts of cocaine, including Switzerland (Hoffman-

LaRoche, CIBA) and the Netherlands. Much smaller amounts of cocaine were also manufactured in Great Britain and France (France was a leading manufacturer of heroin and morphine but never produced substantial amounts of cocaine). For an account of drug production in Europe, see Alan A. Block, "European Drug Traffic and Traffickers between the Wars: The Policy of Suppression and Its Consequences," *Journal of Social History* 23 (Winter 1989): 315–37. Block suggests, quite rightly, that "legitimately" manufactured heroin, morphine, and cocaine remained the main source of supply through the 1920s.

51. According to a May 1908 announcement in the *American Journal of Pharmacy,* C. F. Boehringer & Soehne discontinued its branch house in New York and handed over the distribution of its drugs to Merck. By World War I, Merck may have been the largest single manufacturer of cocaine.

52. A smaller American chemical manufacturer, the Schaefer Alkaloid Works of Maywood, New Jersey, supplied the Coca-Cola Company with its de-cocainized coca leaves.

53. Powers-Weightman-Rosengarten merged with Merck in 1927.

54. Manufacturers often employed endorsements to promote their cocaine. Boehringer included the endorsements of many prominent physicians, including Carl Koller (who had moved to New York by the time of his endorsement) and W. Golden Mortimer. McKesson & Robbins received endorsement of its product from the *British Medical Journal.* Sigmund Freud was persuaded to endorse the quality and purity of Parke, Davis cocaine.

55. The information regarding Mallinckrodt sales and profits comes from a handwritten document dated September 1920, which lists the manufacturing costs, selling price, percentage profit on sales, amount sold in pounds, and gross profits for every one of the company's products; the list is in the Edward Mallinckrodt, Jr. Papers (hereafter EMP), Western Historical Manuscript Collection, University of Missouri, St. Louis, box 49, folder 1050. One reason that cocaine was so profitable is that the selling price exceeded any other Mallinckrodt product, and the mark-up (47.5% for cocaine hydrochloride) exceeded every product except morphine and heroin.

56. H. B. Rosengarten to Hamilton Wright, October 18, 1909, Records of the U.S. Delegations to International Opium Commission and Conferences (hereafter USDIOC), National Archives.

57. John Wyeth & Brothers to Hamilton Wright, October 19, 1909, USDIOC. Even after the government attempted to compel companies to register their imports of coca and cocaine legally, some firms continued to resist. When the Treasury Department created a registration requirement in 1913 (which was replaced shortly thereafter by the Harrison Act), Lehn & Fink defied the order by importing 1,000 ounces of cocaine from Rotterdam the month the requirement went into effect, without declaring its action. Agents of the Bureau of Chemistry in the Department of Agriculture (the predecessor of the Food and Drug Administration) complained that "it is therefore apparent that unless Customs authorities at this port enforce the provisions of the act . . . we will be greatly handicapped in our endeavor to keep importation of this product under surveillance." H. Lind to Chief Inspector, Bureau of Chemistry, October 24, 1913, BC. The Lehn & Fink importation also failed to appear in the weekly record of the *OPDR.*

58. Treasury Department, *Traffic in Narcotic Drugs* (Washington, D.C.: GPO, 1919), 9. It should be noted that other conclusions of this Treasury Department report were wildly inaccurate, including its famous conclusion that there were approximately one million opi-

ate addicts in the United States. Although often repeated, this statistic was a wild exaggeration, as David Courtwright has shown.

59. Richard Ashley, *Cocaine: Its History, Uses, and Effects* (New York: Warner Books, 1976); Joel Phillips and Ronald W. Wynne, *Cocaine: The Mystique and the Reality* (New York: Avon Books, 1980).

60. Charles E. Terry and Mildred Pellens, *Preliminary Report on Studies of the Use of Narcotics under the Provisions of Federal Law in Six Communities* (New York: Bureau of Social Hygiene, 1924), 16–17; Lawrence Kolb and A. G. Du Mez, *The Prevalence and Trend of Drug Addiction in the United States and Factors Influencing It* (Washington, D.C.: GPO, 1924), 16.

61. "Fiftieth Annual Meeting of the Association: Detailed Report of the Proceedings," *American Druggist* 41 (September 1902): 162–64.

Four   Selling Science

1. For consistency, I use the terms *patent medicines* and *patent medicine manufacturers* rather than *proprietaries* and *proprietary manufacturers*.

2. Advertisement in the *Pharmaceutical Era* (December 1, 1898): 10, soliciting orders for the Sixth Edition of the *Era Druggists' Directory*. The states having the most manufacturers included New York (1,623), Pennsylvania (599), and Illinois (502). From the Kremers Reference Files, F. B. Power Pharmaceutical Library, University of Wisconsin–Madison (hereafter KRF).

3. For the history of food and drug legislation before the 1906 act, see Mitchell Okun, *Fair Play in the Marketplace: The First Battle for Pure Food and Drugs* (1986). For the origins of the 1906 act, see James Harvey Young, *Pure Food: Securing the Federal Food and Drug Act of 1906* (Princeton: Princeton University Press, 1990).

4. See Paul Starr, *The Social Transformation of American Medicine* (New York: Basic Books, 1982), especially chap. 3, "The Consolidation of Professional Authority, 1850–1930."

5. See David L. Cowen and William H. Helfand, *Pharmacy: An Illustrated History* (New York: Abrams, 1990).

6. The story of the founding of Parke, Davis & Company is related in Francis E. Stewart to Dr. George H. Simmons, April 18, 1913, Francis Edward Stewart Papers (hereafter SP), MS 606, Archives Division, State Historical Society of Wisconsin, American Institute of the History of Pharmacy Collection.

7. Individuals with experience as physicians or pharmacists included Edward R. Squibb, Wallace Calvin Abbott, John Uri Lloyd, Eli Lilly, and A. R. L. Dohme (of the Baltimore firm Sharp & Dohme).

8. Interview with F. W. Robinson, 1958, 10–11, Parke, Davis & Company Collection, Burton Historical Collection, Detroit Public Library (hereafter PDC); McKesson & Robbins, *Prices Current*.

9. Francis E. Stewart, "Brief History of the Founding of Parke, Davis & Co.'s Scientific Department," SP.

10. Parke, Davis even attempted to buy the financially struggling *Medical and Surgical Reporter* in the mid 1880s, although it was unable to do so. George S. Davis to F. E. Stewart, October 7, 1886, SP.

11. The *Medical Age* was published in Detroit; George S. Davis was listed as the publisher and John J. Mulheron, M.D., as editor.

12. William R. Warner Co., *Coca* (Philadelphia, 1885), 10.

13. George S. Davis, *The Pharmacology of the Newer Materia Medica* (Detroit, 1892). Although published in 1892, advance sheets from this work were prepared and distributed to physicians and pharmacists as they were completed. Examples of these pamphlets may be found in the collections of the Lloyd Library. See, specifically, Drug Price Lists and Circulars, 1870–1970, Collection 101, Lloyd Library and Museum, Cincinnati (hereafter LL).

14. McKesson & Robbins price lists (from the collections of the American Institute of the History of Pharmacy). Note that McKesson & Robbins continued to recommend its cocaine pills for the treatment of the "opium and chloral habits" as late as 1897, although this claim was dropped in the 1901 price list and catalog. The *Oil, Paint, and Drug Reporter* (hereafter *OPDR*) enthusiastically supported Hammond in his disputes with other physicians, especially J. B. Mattison. An 1887 editorial said of Hammond's work, "Here is an open challenge which should be accepted by the defamers of cocaine who have sought to place it in bad repute and cause its burial for good. But the drug is on top and will continue to hold its own and grow in popularity as an anesthetic notwithstanding the opposition of otherwise interested medical men and sensational writers." Editorial, *OPDR* (March 9, 1887).

15. Squibb's comments are reported in Francis E. Stewart to Parke, Davis & Company, December 1, 1879, SP.

16. Francis E. Stewart, "Attack on Parke, Davis and Co.'s New Remedy Business by Their Competitors Led by Dr. Horatio R. Bigelow, of Washington, D.C.," SP. As an illustration of the competition in the ethical pharmaceutical field, forty thousand copies of the article were distributed with advertising donated by competitors. Francis E. Stewart to Dr. George H. Simmons, April 18, 1913, SP.

17. Francis E. Stewart, "Founding of the Scientific Department of Parke, Davis & Co.," SP. John Parascandola, in his recent work on the emergence of American pharmacology, also notes that Parke, Davis established the first industrial laboratory. Parascandola suggests that "the goal of these laboratories was generally not research aimed at the development of new products or innovation in general, but rather the standardization of the quantity and quality of ingredients and the potency of existing products." The Parke, Davis experience with coca and cocaine certainly confirms Parascandola's observation. I would suggest, however, that the scientific staff of Parke, Davis also served to promote the company and its products with physicians. Parascandola himself observes that academic pharmacologists evinced considerable hostility toward their industrial counterparts, suspicious of the combination of science and business. See John Parascandola, *The Development of American Pharmacology: John J. Abel and the Shaping of a Discipline* (Baltimore: Johns Hopkins University Press, 1992), especially chap. 5, "Pharmacologists in Government and Industry."

18. Recognizing the value of name recognition, the firm also hired Horatio C. Wood as editor of the *Therapeutic Gazette* in 1884 or 1885. Wood, one of the leading medical figures in the United States, contributed occasional articles to the publication. George Davis, however, referred to Wood as a "figurehead" who made only a small contribution. George S. Davis to Henry Hurd Rusby, December 21, 1889, SP.

19. While Lyons was employed by Parke, Davis, he wrote several texts on pharmaceutical chemistry, including his *Manual of Practical Pharmaceutical Assaying*, published by Parke, Davis. Lyons was hired away from the Detroit College of Medicine in 1881 and

worked for the company until 1897. Remarkably, Lyons continued to work for another twenty-eight years for rival Nelson, Baker & Co. until his death in 1925. Albert B. Lyons file, KRF.

20. Francis E. Stewart to Robert P. Fischelis, SP. It should not be assumed, however, that the scientists in the employ of Parke, Davis readily misled their colleagues. As Stewart himself wrote, in an angry letter to Parke, Davis, their agreement "obligates you to publish the results of such tests in the *Therapeutic Gazette* whether favorable to the drug tested or otherwise. These reports must contain the truth, the whole truth, and nothing but the truth." Francis E. Stewart to Parke, Davis & Co., January 9, 1883, SP. As for George S. Davis, the financial interests of the business often led him to question the wisdom of the "scientific" approach. Once, when the release of detailed information on one drug had caused Parke, Davis to lose its monopoly, Davis wrote to Stewart, "it does seem at times that those of our staff who assume to themselves the position of advisers to us upon our ethical course are leading us astray through a tortuous channel which abounds in rocks on either side, and that between these rocks of competition and of an unappreciative and hostile medical profession we shall be ground to pieces so far as our interests in any individual article worthy of competition is concerned." George S. Davis to Francis E. Stewart, December 5, 1889, SP.

21. In 1888, Parke, Davis reprinted Rusby's *Therapeutic Gazette* article on coca (which had already reappeared in several national publications) as a pamphlet. See Henry Hurd Rusby, *Coca at Home and Abroad* (Detroit: George S. Davis, 1888), LL.

22. Albert B. Lyons file, KRF.

23. Albert B. Lyons, "The Various Brands of Cocaine Muriate in the Market," *Medical Age* 3 (July 25, 1885): 327–28.

24. Parke, Davis & Company, *Brochures* (*Medical Monographs*), LL.

25. George S. Davis to Francis E. Stewart, June 20, 1885, SP.

26. See for example, Parke, Davis & Company to Francis E. Stewart, April 6, 1885, SP, in which the firm requested that Stewart deliver "samples" of cocaine to Drs. Strawbridge and Morris in Philadelphia. Stewart, although in the employ of Parke, Davis, had his medical practice in Philadelphia. In another letter, Stewart himself made the request on behalf of another physician.

27. Francis E. Stewart, "Coca Leaf Cigars and Cigarettes," *Philadelphia Medical Times* 15 (September 19, 1885): 935.

28. C. N. Anderson, "Memoirs," PDC.

29. Parke, Davis & Company catalog, 1894, 90.

30. C. F. Boehringer & Soehne to Pharmaceutical Publishing Co., August 28, 1896, Boehringer & Soehne file, KRF.

31. Bureau of the Census, *Manufactures 1914*, "Special Reports on Selected Industries."

32. The best known historian of patent medicine quackery is James Harvey Young, whose long career has detailed the persistent strain of health fraud and quackery in American history. His most recent work, *American Health Quackery: Collected Essays by James Harvey Young* (Princeton: Princeton University Press, 1992), summarizes much of this work.

33. The work of J. Worth Estes provides an interesting and important counterpoint to Young's. See particularly J. Worth Estes, "The Pharmacology of Nineteenth Century Patent Medicines," *Pharmacy in History* 30 (1988): 3–18.

34. Monroe Martin King, "Dr. John S. Pemberton: Originator of Coca Cola," *Pharmacy in History* 29 (1987): 85–89; James Harvey Young, "Three Atlanta Pharmacists," *Pharmacy in History* 31 (1989): 16–22; and J. C. Louis and Harvey Z. Yazijian, *The Cola Wars* (New York: Everest House Publishers, 1980).

35. "Coca-Cola a Triumph Over Nature," *National Druggist* (July 1896): 214.

36. "Danger in Imitation Coca-Cola," *National Druggist* (July 1907): 259.

37. Pendergrast discovered the formula while researching the history of Coca-Cola in the company's archives. Although the formula is almost certainly the original, it has been modified since Pemberton's time. See Mark Pendergrast, *For God, Country and Coca-Cola: The Unauthorized History of the Great American Soft Drink and the Company That Makes It* (New York: Charles Scribner's Sons, 1993), 421–25.

38. Richard S. Tedlow, *New and Improved: The Story of Mass Marketing in America* (New York: Basic Books, 1990), 28.

39. Ibid., 29.

40. *Nostrums and Quackery* (Chicago: American Medical Association Press, 1912).

41. Interstate seizure file 8092-a, notice of judgment 594 "Wiseola"; interstate seizure files 19577-a and 8094-a, notice of judgment 202 "Koca Nola"; interstate seizure files 19578-a and 9103-a, notice of judgment 296 "Kos-Kola"; records of the Food and Drug Administration, Rockville, Md. (hereafter FDA).

42. W. Golden Mortimer, *Peru: History of Coca, "The Divine Plant" of the Incas* (New York, 1901).

43. The Lloyd Library has eleven issues of *Mariani's Coca Leaf* from 1903 and 1904 in its collections.

44. Charles N. Crittenton, *Catalogue of Proprietary Medicines and Druggists' Sundries* (1891), 332–33.

45. Advertisement in *Apothecary* (March 1905): 851.

46. Ibid., 61.

47. The Cocarettes advertisement is reprinted in Patricia M. Tice, *Altered States: Alcohol and Other Drugs in America* (Rochester, N.Y.: The Strong Museum, 1992), 49.

48. *Nostrums and Quackery,* 537, 573.

49. G. F. Harvey Company to U.S. Department of Agriculture, June 23, 1914, Bureau of Chemistry (United States Department of Agriculture [hereafter USDA]), RG97, National Archives, Washington, D.C.

50. Waugh's study was also reprinted by the ethical firm, William R. Warner Co. in its monograph "Coca." The Coca-Bola label is reprinted in *Nostrums and Quackery,* 487.

51. Parke, Davis was among the leading promoters of cocaine yet initially did a substantial business in both coca and coca products. In 1885, the firm did the largest share of its business in fluid extract preparations. An 1886 inventory suggests the relative importance of fluid extracts to the company. D. O. Haynes, Superintendent, Parke, Davis & Company to George S. Davis, April 1, 1886, Parke, Davis file, KRF. The value of the firm's fluid extracts ($43,672) represented approximately 32 percent of its entire inventory of manufactured goods, with the stock of solid and gelatine-coated pills the next largest groups (at $18,225 and $14,830, respectively). Fluid extract of coca appears to have become among the most important of these products. An internal memo from 1885 reveals that the firm had a storage capacity of 1,050 pounds of fluid extract coca. The storage capacity of the fourteen other fluid extracts mentioned in the correspondence ranged from 20 to 160

pounds, with most either 20, 24, or 40 pounds. D. O. Haynes to B. R. Finlayson, January 19, 1886, Parke, Davis file, KRF. These estimates of coca and cocaine production synthesize data from several manufacturing reports.

52. In Van Schaack's catalog for 1915, however, only one of these articles was still being sold. Moreover, Mariani's Wine had changed its composition to eliminate all coca and cocaine.

53. *Nostrums and Quackery,* 428–29.

54. Bureau of Chemistry hearing 144, September 4, 1908, interstate seizure file 27, notice of judgment 1077 "Dr. Tucker's Specific for Asthma," box 416, FDA.

55. "Treatment of a 'Bad Cold,'" *National Druggist* (February 1895): 234.

56. *Pharmacal Notes* 1 (1894): 21.

57. *Nostrums and Quackery,* 535.

58. There are three reasons why tests of the same product revealed differing amounts of cocaine. First, the manufacturers of catarrh cures made little effort to standardize their products. Second, the testing and analysis process was itself variable. Finally, some manufacturers of the various catarrh cures reduced the amount of cocaine in their product in an effort to meet the requirements of various state laws passed after 1900.

59. Harry N. Pringle, Christian Civic League to Hamilton Wright, December 3, 1909, U.S. Delegation to International Opium Commission and Conferences.

60. *Nostrums and Quackery,* 551.

61. Samuel Hopkins Adams, *The Great American Fraud* (Chicago, 1912), 178. The AMA reprinted Adams' *Collier's* series in this volume. The Cole's circular was originally published in the June 8, 1907 issue of *Collier's.*

62. Bureau of Chemistry to Attorney General, March 21, 1910, interstate seizure file 9673-b, notice of judgment 727 "Az-Ma-Syde," box 240, FDA.

63. Interstate seizure file 9164-a, notice of judgment 323 "Remedy For Hay Fever and Catarrh," box 230, FDA.

64. Ibid.

Five   The Transformation of Cocaine Use

1. W. Sheppegrell, "The Abuse and Dangers of Cocain," *Medical News* 73 (October 1, 1898): 421–22.

2. Ibid.

3. T. D. Crothers, "Cocaine-Inebriety," *Quarterly Journal of Inebriety* 20 (1898): 370.

4. John Uri Lloyd, *A Treatise on Coca (Erythroxylon Coca): "The Divine Plant of the Incas"* (Cincinnati, 1913), 4.

5. Reprinted in Angelo Mariani, *Coca Erythroxylon (Vin Mariani): Its Uses in the Treatment of Disease,* 4th ed. (New York, 1886), 39.

6. For a comprehensive look at the world of the roustabout, see Eric Arnesen, *Waterfront Workers of New Orleans: Race, Class, and Politics, 1863–1923* (New York: Oxford University Press, 1991). Another useful work is Daniel Rosenberg, *New Orleans Dockworkers: Race, Labor, and Unionism, 1892–1923* (Albany: State University of New York Press, 1988) and, more generally, David Montgomery, *The Fall of the House of Labor: The Workplace, the State, and American Labor Activism, 1865–1925* (New York: Cambridge University Press, 1987), especially chap. 2, "The Common Laborer."

7. "Negro Cocaine Fiends," *Medical News* 81 (November 8, 1902): 895.

8. Q. W. Hunter, "The Evils of Cocaine," *Medical Age* 24 (1906): 331–38.

9. Montgomery, *Fall of the House of Labor,* 96–100.

10. Harris Dickson to Hamilton Wright, December 7, 1909, U.S. Delegation to International Opium Commission and Conferences (hereafter USDIOC).

11. Numerous historical works deal with the question of agricultural labor in the New South. The best overview of the subject is Edward L. Ayers, *The Promise of the New South: Life After Reconstruction* (New York: Oxford University Press, 1992).

12. "Negro Cocaine Fiends," 895.

13. "Negro Cocaine Evil," *New York Times* (March 20, 1905): 14; in 1902, the *Medical News* reported that the operator of a whisky-running ship was also distributing cocaine among the plantations of Mississippi's Yazoo River delta as well as along the lower Mississippi.

14. C. P. Ambler, "Cocaine: Its Uses and Abuses," *Cleveland Medical Gazette* 10 (1894–95): 54–62.

15. Henry O. Whiteside, "The Drug Habit in Nineteenth-century Colorado," *Colorado Magazine* 55 (1978): 47–68.

16. In the winter of 1896–97, the collective cocaine use in the town of Manchester became the subject of national notoriety. Perhaps the greatest publicity came in a series of articles in the *New York Herald*. Beginning in December 1896, the *Herald* reported on the town "mad for cocaine." Choosing a theme often repeated in subsequent years, the *Herald* suggested that the recent efforts by the town to close its saloons and go "dry" had created a cocaine epidemic. See, for example, *New York Herald,* December 28–29, 1896, and January 3, 1897. For other published views of the Manchester experience, see "The Cocaine Habit," *Practical Druggist and Review of Reviews* 1 (March 1897): 36 and T. D. Crothers, "Cocainism," *Quarterly Journal of Inebriety* 32 (1910): 78–84. On the use of cocaine in Maine factories, see Harry N. Pringle, Christian Civic League, to Hamilton Wright, December 3, 1909, USDIOC.

17. Thomas G. Simonton, "The Increase of the Use of Cocaine among the Laity of Pittsburgh," *Philadelphia Medical Journal* 11 (March 28, 1903): 556–60.

18. David Courtwright, recounting the use of cocaine among stevedores, notes that "whether these stevedores took to cocaine on their own initiative, or whether they were introduced to the drug by their foremen, is not known." Courtwright, "The Hidden Epidemic: Opiate Addiction and Cocaine Use in the South, 1860–1920," *Journal of Southern History* 49 (February 1983): 68.

19. Harris Dickson to Wright, USDIOC.

20. Haywood quoted in Page Smith, *America Enters the World: A People's History of the Progressive Era and World War I* (New York: Penguin Books, 1985), 113. Haywood's inclusion of opiates is probably due to his experiences in the West, where employers stocked opiates and cocaine. In the South, cocaine was used more exclusively. For Haywood's travels, see Melvyn Dubofsky, *"Big Bill" Haywood* (New York: St. Martin's Press, 1987).

21. William Ivy Hair, *Carnival of Fury: Robert Charles and the New Orleans Race Riot of 1900* (Baton Rouge: Louisiana State University Press, 1976), 76–77.

22. "Cocaine Debauchery in the South," *American Druggist* 37 (December 24, 1900): 385; "Grand Jury Gets Behind Cocaine Sellers," New Orleans newspaper clipping (ca. October 1910), "Louisiana" file, USDIOC.

23. W. Schweckhardt, "Cocaine in Texas," *American Druggist* (June 7, 1894): 301–2; the popular use of cocaine in 1894 was sufficiently unfamiliar to the editors of the *American Druggist* that they suggested editorially that their correspondent was probably exaggerating the extent of the problem in Dallas.

24. "Cocaine Alley," *American Druggist* 37 (December 10, 1900): 337.

25. "Cocaine Debauchery in the South," 385.

26. Edward Huntington Williams, "The Drug Habit Menace in the South," *Medical Record* 85 (February 7, 1914): 247–49.

27. For an interesting examination of the "new generation," see Howard N. Rabinowitz, *Race Relations in the Urban South, 1865–1890* (New York: Oxford University Press, 1978).

28. "Cocaine Debauchery in the South," 385.

29. Joel Williamson, *A Rage for Order: Black/White Relations in the American South since Emancipation* (New York: Oxford University Press, 1986) offers a valuable look at black images in white society.

30. F. C. Pappe, "Habitual Use of Narcotics," *Midland Druggist* 4 (1902): 632.

31. Lester Grinspoon and James B. Bakalar, *Cocaine: A Drug and Its Social Evolution* (New York: Basic Books, 1976).

32. David Courtwright has worked on this problem and also concludes that "it is fair to say that cocaine was relatively popular in black communities, and that many blacks made at least occasional use of the drug as a euphoric agent." Among the evidence Courtwright provides is Charles Terry's study of cocaine users in Jacksonville, where the rate of cocaine use for blacks was 2.98 per thousand versus 1.61 for white users. Courtwright, *Dark Paradise: Opiate Addiction in America before 1940* (Cambridge: Harvard University Press, 1982). Significantly, cocaine use by blacks was frequently commented on in Northern cities as well. In Baltimore, for example, one account warned that "the habit has grown to an alarming extent, especially among the ignorant and vicious negroes." Hamilton Wright's 1909 survey of police chiefs was especially interesting in this respect. Asked "what classes of the community" were most addicted to cocaine, respondents from around the country indicated blacks as being most inclined toward cocaine use. Cities represented included Spokane, Washington; Jersey City, New Jersey; Cincinnati; Omaha, Nebraska; Charleston, South Carolina; and Providence, Rhode Island. The police chief of Pittsburgh suggested to Wright that fully 90 percent of cocaine users in his city were black, most of the remainder being white denizens of the city's tenderloin. That so many replies agreed on this point proves little, of course — they could as easily reflect selective information, filtered through common racial prejudices.

33. Courtwright, *Dark Paradise*.

34. Charles W. Collins and John Day, "Dope, the New Vice," *Everyday Life* 4 (September 1909): 4–5.

35. Simonton, "Increase of the Use of Cocaine," 556.

36. Alice Hamilton, *Exploring the Dangerous Trades* (Boston: Little, Brown & Co., 1943).

37. C. Moffett, "Rx Cocaine," *Hampton's Magazine* 26 (1911): 595–606; Harvey W. Wiley and Anne L. Pierce, "The Cocaine Crime," *Good Housekeeping* 58 (1914): 393–98.

38. See, for example, "The Sale of Cocaine," *Canadian Pharmaceutical Journal* 42 (1908): 176–77.

39. "Boys Who Use Cocaine," *Pharmaceutical Era* (December 8, 1904): 586.

40. Collins and Day, "Dope, the New Vice," 4.

41. Hamilton Wright, "New York Notes," USDIOC.

42. *Proceedings of the American Pharmaceutical Association* 51 (1903): 476; a 1918 study of drug-addicted draftees at Camp Upton, New York, reported that "eighty percent admitted they were introduced to drugs, by their friends, their friends very largely being immoral women." Charles E. Terry and Mildred Pellens, *The Opium Problem* (New York: Bureau of Social Hygiene, 1918), 120; Wright, "New York Notes," USDIOC.

43. *Proceedings of the American Pharmaceutical Association* 51 (1903): 476.

44. "Snuffing Out the Cocaine Fiend," *Charities and the Commons* 18 (1907): 73.

45. "The Latest Drug Danger," *World's Work* 18 (August 1909): 11869–70.

46. Frederic Poole to Hamilton Wright, 1908, USDIOC; see also, "Cocaine Sales Continue in Tenderloin District," *American Druggist* 51 (October 28, 1907): 320.

47. S. Solis Cohen to Hamilton Wright, 1908, USDIOC.

48. H. P. Hynson, "Report of Committee on Acquirement of the Drug Habit," *National Druggist* (December 1902): 366–68. The report was originally presented to the Pennsylvania Pharmaceutical Association in June 1902.

49. Bingham Dai, *Opium Addiction in Chicago* (reprint, Montclair, N.J.: Patterson Smith, 1970), 111–12.

50. W. T. Neely to Hamilton Wright, July 25, 1908, USDIOC. Historian Jim Baumohl has researched drug use in San Francisco and suggests that legal pressure on opium smokers led many to adopt the hypodermic use of morphine. Baumohl's emphasis on pre-Harrison drug switching as a consequence of law enforcement underscores the importance of regulatory activity in this era and certainly could be extended to include cocaine as well. See Jim Baumohl, "The 'Dope Fiend's Paradise' Revisited: Notes from Research in Progress on Drug Law Enforcement in San Francisco, 1875–1915," *Surveyor* 24 (June 1992): 9.

51. American Pharmaceutical Association, *Report of Committee on Acquirement of Drug Habits* (Baltimore: American Pharmaceutical Association, 1903), 473.

52. *Statistical Report of the Last One Thousand Opium Cases Applying for Treatment at the Keeley Institute* (Dwight, Ill.: Leslie E. Keeley Company, 1899), 8–9, USDIOC. See also Leslie E. Keeley Co. to Hamilton Wright, October 13, 1909, USDIOC.

53. The New York City clinic information is cited in Hans W. Maier, *Der Kokainismus,* trans. Oriana Josseau Kalant (Toronto: Addiction Research Foundation, 1987).

54. By way of comparison, Lawrence Kolb initiated a study of "addicts who were addicted by the prescribing of an opiate for self-medication for a disease and became addicted because of it." Kolb wanted no pleasure users in this study: "persons who became addicted to opium because of the influence of associates, by smoking, for the thrill of it or for other inexcusable reasons (the so-called dissipated underworld addicts) are of no interest for the purpose of this study." Of the 150 medically addicted opiate addicts Kolb surveyed, only nine had ever used cocaine, and none was apparently still using cocaine. This is in marked contrast to Kolb's other survey of addicts, representing a wider array of drug-using careers — approximately 45 percent of whom had used cocaine (about 9% were *current* opiate/cocaine users).

55. David Courtwright has made the case that the popularization of heroin must be understood in the context of the increasing difficulty of obtaining cocaine.

56. "New Danger from Use of Heroin," *American Druggist* (May 1913): 21–22.

57. Fred V. Williams, *The Hop-Heads: Personal Experiences among the Users of 'Dope' in the San Francisco Underworld* (San Francisco, 1920).

58. In addition to the vast anecdotal evidence, a number of social and medical studies, although problematic, also suggest that cocaine users were becoming younger. The average ages of addicts in unpublished manuscript case histories collected by Lawrence Kolb indicated that cocaine addicts tended to be relatively younger than the addict population as a whole. The average age, by current drug of addiction, was: morphine, 40.2 years; heroin 30.4 years; opiate/cocaine 28.8 years; and cocaine, 25.6 years. A number of other studies also examined the age of addiction. Table N.1 shows the results of a survey of drug addicts committed to San Quentin Penitentiary; the survey revealed that drug use was rarely initiated before age 16 or after age 25.

59. Charles E. Terry and Mildred Pellens, *Preliminary Report on Studies of the Use of Narcotics under the Provisions of Federal Law in Six Communities* (New York, 1924), 115.

60. Kolb's unpublished addict studies (see Note 54) bear a striking similarity to the McIver and Price data. Kolb categorized origins as either through associations, physicians, self-medication, or unknown (Table N.2).

61. Collins and Day, "Dope, The New Vice," 4.

62. Martin I. Wilbert, "The Number and Kind of Drug Addicts," *Public Health Reports,* vol. 30 (Washington, D.C.: GPO, 1915).

63. Herbert William Powers, "Morphin and Cocain Addiction with Special Reference To Prognosis," *Illinois Medical Journal* 27 (1915): 441–43.

64. *Limiting Production of Habit-Forming Drugs and Raw Materials from Which They Are Made: Hearings before the Committee on Foreign Affairs,* 67th Cong., 4th sess., 1923, 55–56.

65. John C. Burnham, *Bad Habits: Drinking, Smoking, Taking Drugs, Gambling, Sexual Misbehavior, and Swearing in American History* (New York: New York University Press, 1993), chap. 5, "Taking Drugs." Burnham argues that a fundamental shift occurred in the late nineteenth and early twentieth centuries. Drug taking, which had previously borne little stigma or social sanction, was redirected in nonmedical ways by users who consciously adopted a deviant identity. Cocaine, according to Burnham, "illustrates this transformation to deviancy" (p. 118). Burnham recognizes that users, rather than laws, were largely re-

TABLE N.1
Age at Initiation of Drug Use Among Addicts at San Quentin Penitentiary

Age at Drug Initiation	No. of Addicts
8–15	6
16–20	48
21–25	24
25–30	12
30–40	12
40+	0

SOURCE: L. L. Stanley, "Morphinism and Crime," *Journal of the American Institute of Criminal Law and Criminology* 8 (May 1917–March 1918): 750–51.

TABLE N.2
Origins of Addiction

Origins	Morphine	Heroin	Combined	Cocaine	Other	Totals
Associations	23.6% (21)	71.4% (45)	81.3% (13)	100% (7)	0.0% (0)	47.8% (86
Physician	33.7% (30)	11.1% (7)	6.3% (1)	0.0% (0)	20.0% (1)	21.7% (39
Self-medication	38.2% (34)	15.9% (10)	6.3% (1)	0.0% (0)	80.0% (4)	27.2% (49
Unknown	4.5% (4)	1.6% (1)	6.3% (1)	0.0% (0)	0.0% (0)	3.3% (6
TOTALS	100% (89)	100% (63)	100.2% (16)	100% (7)	100% (5)	100% (180

SOURCE: Manuscript records of addict case histories, Lawrence Kolb Papers, Box 6, National Library of Medicine, History c Medicine Division, Washington, D.C.

sponsible for this important shift. The federal Harrison Act, according to Burnham, "only ratified the shift away from middle-class status" (p. 117). This argument, of course, owes much to Courtwright, *Dark Paradise.*

66. Indeed, the author of a study of drug addicts at Bellevue Hospital was one of many to use precisely these terms: "the great majority [of addicts] take their first step through being unfortunate enough to meet and associate with addicts . . . this is particularly true of the large centers of population, and there can be no doubt that overcrowding, congestion, insanitary surroundings, and a lack of the facilities for healthful recreation are predisposing factors in drug addiction. Under these circumstances a drug addict becomes a focus of infection, as it were, and through contact with susceptible individuals serves to spread the evil. With this sort of environment the drug habit is considered to be highly contagious, particularly among minors." W. A. Bloedorn, "Studies of Drug Addicts," *U.S. Naval Medical Bulletin* 11 (1917); cited in Terry and Pellens, *The Opium Problem,* 117.

67. "Public Waking Up to Cocaine Menace," *New York Times* (August 3, 1908): 5.

Six   Private Acts, Public Concerns

1. Charles H. Leichliter, "Fighting the Demon Cocaine," *Sunday Record-Herald* (November 29, 1908): 5.

2. The characterization of the nineteenth century as a "dope fiend's paradise" figured prominently in Edward Brecher's widely cited study, *Licit and Illicit Drugs* (Boston: Little, Brown & Co., 1972).

3. Leichliter, "Fighting the Demon Cocaine," 5.

4. George William Norris, "A Case of Cocain Habit of Ten Months Duration Treated by Complete and Immediate Withdrawal of the Drug," *Philadelphia Medical Journal* 7 (February 9, 1901): 304.

5. Stephen Lett, "Cocaine Addiction and Its Diagnosis," *Canada Lancet* 31 (December 1898): 830.

6. Assistant Chief Resident Physician, Philadelphia General Hospital to Hamilton Wright, December 1, 1908, U.S. Delegation to International Opium Commission and Conferences (hereafter USDIOC).

7. C. W. Boynge to Hamilton Wright, August 12, 1908, USDIOC.

8. N.S. Yawger, "Cocain Intoxication," *New York Medical Journal* 92 (December 3, 1910): 1132.

9. "Cocaine Victims in Torture," *New York Times* (September 15, 1908).

10. "Boy Cocaine Snuffers Hunted by the Police," *New York Times* (January 8, 1907) 6: 3.

11. Chicago Civil Service Commission, *Final Report: Civil Service Commission, City of Chicago Police Investigation, 1911–1912* (reprint, New York: Arno Press, 1971), 24.

12. "Go After Dope Sellers," *Syracuse Herald* (June 21, 1906): Section C46 (i) I, Kremers Reference Files, F. B. Power Pharmaceutical Library, University of Wisconsin–Madison (hereafter KRF).

13. "Victim of Cocaine Prays for Relief," *Syracuse Journal* (June 21, 1906): Section C46 (i) I, KRF.

14. Ibid., n.p.

15. "George Thorpe Would Stop Sale of Cocaine," *Syracuse Standard* (June 22, 1906): Section C46 (g) IV, KRF.

16. Yawger, "Cocain Intoxication," 1132. A "marasmic" condition referred to a wasting away of the patient, including emaciation and severe weight loss.

17. Charles W. Collins and John Day, "Dope, the New Vice," *Everyday Life* (September 1909): 4.

18. Ibid.

19. Thomas G. Simonton, "The Increase of the Use of Cocaine among the Laity of Pittsburgh," *Philadelphia Medical Journal* 11 (March 28, 1903): 557.

20. Charles B. Whilden, California State Board of Pharmacy to Hamilton Wright, September 17, 1908, USDIOC.

21. Arthur Woods, *Dangerous Drugs: The World Fight against Illicit Traffic in Narcotics* (New Haven: Yale University Press, 1931), 29–30; N. S. Yawger observed that those who ceased the use of the drug never ceased the craving for it. Yawger concluded that "a permanent cure is extraordinarily rare."

22. As Jim Baumohl has observed in his study of early drug law enforcement in San Francisco, that city's Cubic Air Ordinance and vagrancy laws were both used as part of a "highly selective pattern of enforcement laid first on Chinese opium smokers and white fellow-travelers, then on impoverished white morphine addicts, and then on working-class white opium smokers who observed the color line." Baumohl suggests that these campaigns "intensified" by the 1870s and continued through the passage of the Harrison Act. Jim Baumohl, "The 'Dope Fiend's Paradise' Revisited: Notes from Research in Progress on Drug Law Enforcement in San Francisco, 1875–1915," *Surveyor* (June 1992): 3–12.

23. Thomas A. McQuaide to Hamilton Wright, June 29, 1909, USDIOC.

24. Chicago Civil Service Commission, *Final Report,* 24.

25. Inspector Edward McCann to Hamilton Wright, August 11, 1908, USDIOC.

26. "Boy Cocaine Snuffers Hunted by the Police," 6:3.

27. "Report of the Committee on the Drug Evil," *Proceedings of the Thirteenth Annual Conference of the New York State Association of Magistrates* (1922); reprint, Charles E. Terry and Mildred Pellens, *Preliminary Report on Studies of the Use of Narcotics under the Provisions of Federal Law in Six Communities* (New York, 1924), 853–60.

28. *Annual Report of the Board of Police Commissioners,* 1911, 1914.

29. Arthur D. Layne, Sergeant of Police, to Thomas S. Duke, Captain of Police, June 26, 1909, USDIOC.

30. Chicago Civil Service Commission, *Final Report,* 27.

31. Hamilton Wright, "New York Notes," USDIOC.

32. Whilden to Wright, USDIOC. Whilden also observed that most drug users from the "criminal or prostitute class" who received any kind of extended treatment did so in one of the five state hospitals for the insane. Whilden reported, however, that "in the asylums the majority of those committed are from the better class of society."

33. American Pharmaceutical Association, *Report of Committee on Acquirement of Drug Habits* (Baltimore: American Pharmaceutical Association, 1903), 473.

34. W. A. Doyle to Hamilton Wright, June 23, 1909, USDIOC.

35. J. T. Sullivan to Hamilton Wright, June 22, 1909, USDIOC.

36. This category corresponds roughly to the model of the drugs/crime relationship articulated by Paul Goldstein in 1990. Goldstein classified drug-related homicides into three general categories: (1) economic-compulsive: crime committed by users for the purposes of obtaining resources to purchase drugs; (2) systemic: crime associated with the business and control of drug distribution; and (3) psychopharmacological: activity directly caused by the effects of the drug itself. The small amount of crime and violence directly associated with cocaine selling (what Goldstein calls *systemic* violence) will be considered in chapter 6. See Paul J. Goldstein, "Drugs and Violent Crime," in *Violence: Patterns, Causes, Public Policy*, ed. Neil Alan Weiner, Margaret A. Zahn, and Rita J. Sagi (San Diego: Harcourt Brace Jovanovich, 1990), 295–303.

37. Alice Hamilton, *Exploring the Dangerous Trades* (Boston: Little, Brown & Co., 1943).

38. One of the earliest reports of chronic catarrh cure use appeared in the June 1897 *JAMA,* and it suggests how expensive such use could be. The journal reported the case of a woman who had been using three bottles of catarrh snuff each week for several months. Because each bottle contained 80 grains of snuff with 1.75 percent cocaine, the woman's weekly consumption of cocaine was approximately 4.2 grains. The price of each bottle was at least 50¢, whereas 4.2 grains of cocaine could probably have been purchased alone for no more than 15¢, or 10 percent of the price of the catarrh cures.

39. Q. W. Hunter, "The Evils of Cocaine," *Medical Age* 24 (1906): 336.

40. Jim Baumohl has effectively shown that the same financial strain and corresponding criminality applied to morphine addicts in pre–Harrison Act San Francisco. Baumohl writes, "A modest [morphine] habit requiring from $1.25 to $1.75 per week could be demanding indeed; a large habit could be disastrous. Even if we take into account the fact that criminal careers often precede addiction, we must acknowledge the extreme economic pressures on working and lower-class addicts. The 'dope fiend's paradise' scenario ignores this intersection of addiction and material deprivation." Baumohl, "The 'Dope Fiend's Paradise' Revisited," 8–9.

41. Heine Marks, "The General Treatment of Habitual and Periodic Alcoholic, Morphine, and Cocaine Inebriates," *Quarterly Journal of Inebriety* 18 (1896): 148.

42. David F. Musto, "Illicit Price of Cocaine in Two Eras: 1908–1914 and 1982–1989," *Connecticut Medicine* 54 (1990): 321–26.

43. *Western Pennsylvania Retail Druggist* (hereafter *WPRD*) (January 1914): 13; *WPRD* (June 1914): 10; *WPRD* (July 1914): 8. Drug wholesalers and manufacturers found their supplies of cocaine the subject of continual pilfering, so much so that drug clerks and other employees often became an important part of local cocaine distribution.

44. J. B. Cook, chief of police, city of San Francisco, to Hamilton Wright, July 5, 1909; J. Grant Long, office of the chief of police, city of Wilkes-Barre, Pennsylvania, to Wright,

June 25, 1909; and Fred Kohler, chief of police, Cleveland, Ohio, to Wright, June 9, 1909, USDIOC.

45. It should be noted that Lewis' opposition was reinforced by his belief in a variation of the theories of Cesare Lombroso, that "the causes of criminal conduct are most usually found in the physical and mental makeup of the criminal himself." Such a view was hard to reconcile with the view that drugs inspired criminal behavior. New York City Mayor's Committee on Public Welfare, *Minutes of the First Meeting,* May 29, 1919, Copeland Papers, Michigan Historical Collections, Bentley Historical Library, University of Michigan.

46. Ibid.

47. Ibid.

48. T. D. Crothers, "Cocainism," *Quarterly Journal of Inebriety* 32 (1910): 78–84.

49. William Healy, *The Individual Delinquent: A Text-Book of Diagnosis and Prognosis for All Concerned in Understanding Offenders* (Boston: Little, Brown & Co., 1915), 275–78.

50. Healy wrote, for example, that cocaine "induces unwonted boldness on the part of weak individuals," a characteristic that he believed Case 29 fully exhibited. But what of the connections to criminal behavior and to venereal disease? Here Healy's case study failed to offer a persuasive explanation for linking them with cocaine use.

51. J. B. Mattison, "Cocainism," *Medical Record* 43 (1893): 34–36.

52. Edward Huntington Williams, "The Drug Habit Menace in the South," *Medical Record* 85 (February 7, 1914): 247.

53. Ibid., 248.

54. Ibid., 247.

55. William Ivy Hair, *Carnival of Fury: Robert Charles and the New Orleans Race Riot of 1900* (Baton Rouge: Louisiana State University Press, 1976), 132.

56. *New York Herald* (September 29, 1913). E. H. Williams also cited this incident as an example of the kinds of actions one might expect from "the cocainized negro."

57. Joel Williamson, *A Rage for Order: Black/White Relations in the American South since Emancipation* (New York: Oxford University Press, 1986), 142.

58. Hunter, "The Evils of Cocaine," 331–38.

59. "Aaron Martin Sold 470 Ounces of Cocaine in Nine Months," *New Orleans Item,* KRF. The cocaine/violence connection was well publicized in journalistic explorations of the drug problem. Charles Collins' series in *Everyday Life* spoke urgently of the cocaine problem in Chicago, describing the exploits of "cocainized 'jack-rollers' "; young men who "in many cases . . . have beaten their helpless victims to death." Collins viewed cocaine as a direct cause of the violence: "the professional 'crook' or the redoubtable 'yeggman' draws his revolver only as a last resort, but the cocaine fiend, usually nothing more than a cheap pickpocket or small thief, will blaze away as if celebrating the Fourth of July at the slightest excuse." Collins and Day, "Dope, The New Vice," 5.

Seven   The Cautionary Tale

1. J. L. Lynch, Food and Drug Inspector, to W. G. Campbell, Chief Inspector, December 21, 1909, "Coca-Cola" file, Food and Drug Administration (hereafter FDA).

2. Samuel Hopkins Adams, *The Great American Fraud* (Chicago, 1912), 44.

3. Nathan S. Davis, "Effect of Proprietary Literature on Medical Men," *JAMA* 46 (May 5, 1906): 1339, in Harry Milton Marks, "Ideas as Reforms: Therapeutic Experiments and

Medical Practice, 1900–1980" (Ph.D. diss., Massachusetts Institute of Technology, 1987), 31. Marks makes the observation that the combined demand for "rational therapeutics" — the application of drugs based upon laboratory experimentation — and desire to consolidate medical authority led to the establishment of regulatory agencies in the early twentieth century. It seems likely that the medical profession's experience with cocaine was part of their collective experience, which suggested the need for regulation and control. It is ironic, though, that many of the earliest cocaine enthusiasts had been from the ranks of supporters of laboratory experimentation and had pronounced cocaine a successful product of such work.

4. Lewis D. Mason, "Patent and Proprietary Medicines as the Cause of the Alcohol and Opium Habit or Other Forms of Narcomania — With Some Suggestions as to How the Evil May Be Remedied," *Quarterly Journal of Inebriety* 25 (January 1903): 6.

5. Ibid., 8–9.

6. *United States v Mayfield, Bradley, Hawkins, and Altman,* District Court, N.D. Alabama, district court case 1679. The trial transcript is in the "Coca-Cola" file, FDA; see also interstate seizure file 8090-a, notice of judgment 326 "Celery-Cola," box 230, FDA.

7. "Cocaine in United States," *Canadian Pharmaceutical Journal* 42 (1909): 396.

8. Adams, *The Great American Fraud,* 178–79.

9. U.S. Department of Agriculture (hereafter USDA), Bureau of Chemistry (hereafter BC), hearing 972 (January 16, 1912), BC.

10. *The Propaganda for Reform in Proprietary Medicines* (Chicago, American Medical Association), 114–18.

11. For an interesting account of Wiley's battle with Coca-Cola, particularly over caffeine, see Ludy T. Benjamin, Anne M. Rogers, and Angela Rosenbaum, "Coca-Cola, Caffeine, and Mental Deficiency: Harry Hollingworth and the Chattanooga Trial of 1911," *Journal of the History of the Behavioral Sciences* 27 (January 1991): 42–54.

12. "The Celery-Cola Case," interstate seizure file 8090-a, notice of judgment 326 "Celery-Cola," box 230, FDA.

13. Celery-Cola trial transcript, 22.

14. The importance of public opinion may be gauged by another letter written to the Bureau of Chemistry by the Celery-Cola Company in which they pleaded with the government not to release the assay results of one of its other soft drinks: "PEPSIN-OLA is dead. The manufacture of it was long since discontinued, but as the association of the name of the Celery-Cola Co. in connection with the publication of the assay would work us serious injury, we pray that you will not resurrect the remains for this intended post-mortem." J. H. Van Deusen, Celery-Cola Company to the Bureau of Chemistry, June 1, 1909, interstate seizure file 8090-a, notice of judgment 326 "Celery-Cola," box 230, FDA. Whether Pepsin-Ola contained cocaine is not clear, although it seems likely that it did. The government appears to have agreed to the company's request because this product does not appear in the public record.

15. "The Celery-Cola Case," 2–3.

16. Interstate seizure files 16578-a and 31622-a, notice of judgment 694 "Alleged Drug-Habit Cure," FDA.

17. The film was entitled "For His Sons" and was directed by Griffith. The plot revolved around the father's development of a drink called Dopo-Kola. The tragic element to the plot was the son's subsequent addiction to cocaine through consumption of the beverage.

18. J. Leyden White, "The Coca-Cola 'Joker' in the Harrison Narcotic Law," April 29, 1916. RG 90, records of the U.S. Public Health Service (hereafter USPHS), general files "1924–1935," box 66.

19. Wiseola's claim was printed on the company's letterhead; interstate seizure file 8092-a, notice of judgment 594 "Wiseola," box 230, FDA.

20. J. L. Lynch, drug inspector, to W. G. Campbell, chief inspector, November 18, 1910, "Coca-Cola" file, FDA.

21. Nelson, Baker & Company to Arthur E. Paul, "Comments of Dr. A. B. Lyons," January 15, 1926, BC.

22. H. K. Mulford to Francis E. Stewart, Philadelphia, Penn., August 15, 1904; H. K. Mulford to Francis E. Stewart, East Orange, N.J., February 13, 1906, Francis E. Stewart Papers (hereafter SP), Archives Division, State Historical Society of Wisconsin, American Institute of the History of Pharmacy Collection.

23. There are relatively few comprehensive studies of the development of the American pharmaceutical industry in this era. Recent years, however, have seen the publication of several excellent works, including Jonathan Liebenau, *Medical Science and Medical Industry: The Formation of the American Pharmaceutical Industry* (Baltimore: The Johns Hopkins University Press, 1987) and John P. Swann, *Academic Scientists and the Pharmaceutical Industry: Cooperative Research in Twentieth-Century America* (Baltimore: The Johns Hopkins University Press, 1988).

24. *Pharmacal Notes* (February 1896): 2, Parke, Davis & Company Collection (hereafter PDC), Burton Historical Collection, Detroit Public Library.

25. Henry Hurd Rusby, *Jungle Memories* (New York, 1933), 343.

26. The experience of Parke, Davis & Company with Chloretone was itself something of a disaster. Not long after the company began advertising its new product, Chloretone was roundly criticized for being unsafe and ineffective. The Parke, Davis London manager F. M. Fiske wrote in 1901 to Detroit that "complaints re failure of Chloretone as a local anesthetic are coming in thick and fast." Fiske reported comments from physicians such as "entirely displeased" and "absolutely worthless" and stated the obvious in concluding, "it is getting a very black eye right now." Parke, Davis & Company, "Specialties," August 1900–March 1901, PDC. H. K. Mulford, in his private correspondence with former Parke, Davis medical consultant Francis E. Stewart, observed that "we have known for six years that this product was dangerous, that it is simply an old preparation that was put on the shelves and rechristened, the whole matter was faked from the beginning." H. K. Mulford to Francis E. Stewart, October 16, 1905, SP. Exactly what "old preparation" Chloretone was is unclear, but there is no question that Parke, Davis was anxious to forget the entire experience.

27. Parke, Davis hypodermic tablet department, experiments with cocaine, strychnine, and nitroglycerine tablets, April 4, 1899, PDC.

28. Parke, Davis hypodermic tablet department, control department memo, January 15, 1907, PDC; control department memo, October 17, 1907, PDC; control department memo, January 15, 1909, PDC; Francis to Dr. Marshall, January 26, 1907, PDC.

29. *Oil, Paint, and Drug Reporter* (hereafter *OPDR*) (May 4, 1893): 30.

30. Advertisement in *OPDR* (December 16, 1909): 4. Eventually, even Parke, Davis marketed a synthetic cocaine substitute under the trade name Apothesine.

31. In 1893, company superintendent Leon Fink asked the scientific department to provide equivalences for coca and cocaine: "we frequently have occasion to substitute Cocaine

Hydrochloride for Coca leaves in various pharmaceuticals." Leon Fink to Thompson, July 7, 1893, "Specialties," box 3, PDC. For the product formulas, see G. A. Burnham to Leon Fink, November 13, 1896, box 3, PDC; for product deletions, see J. M. Francis, "Memorandum," July 17, 1912, "Solid Extracts and Powdered Extracts," box 28, PDC and also control department memo, November 11, 1907, "Elixirs, Wines and Syrups," box 16, PDC.

32. Lyman F. Kebler, *Habit-Forming Agents: Their Indiscriminate Sale and Use a Menace to the Public Welfare,* USDA Farmer's Bulletin 393 (Washington, D.C.: GPO, 1910), 10.

33. O. W. Smith to Parke, Davis & Company, December 4, 1909, box 20, PDC. In an earlier memorandum, the company's Detroit counsel had been asked whether cocaine laws would "affect all preparations containing Cocaine including" those products "which would not be used by cocaine habitués?" Counsel Woodruff's discouraging reply suggested that they would. Norvell to Counsel Woodruff, memorandum, September 30, 1909, and Woodruff to Norvell, September 30, 1909, box 20, PDC.

34. Bureau of Chemistry hearing 144 "Nathan Tucker's Asthma Specific" (September 4, 1908), BC.

35. The source of the controversy had been the Maltine Company's use of the likenesses of prominent physicians on an 1894 advertising calendar. One of the physicians was Nathan S. Davis, future member of the AMA Council on Pharmacy and Chemistry, who protested that he had "never prescribed an ounce of Maltine, nor written a line concerning it in my life." Davis wrote an angry letter to *JAMA,* which in turn printed Maltine's response.

36. Charles L. Huisking, *Herbs to Hormones: The Evolution of Drugs and Chemicals That Revolutionized Medicine* (Essex, Conn.: Pequot Press, 1968), 68–69.

37. Bureau of Chemistry hearing 64 "Maltine Coca Wine" (November 12, 1907), BC.

38. The Wiseola Company to USDA, May 29, 1909, interstate seizure file 8092-a, notice of judgment 594 "Wiseola," box 230, FDA.

39. General Manager's manifold letter 73, September 29, 1910, box 20, PDC. This letter should not be taken to mean, however, that Parke, Davis was unwilling to *sell* fluid extract of coca, only that it would not protect its customers afterward! The general manager went on to advise company staff that "anything we market is sold for lawful purposes only, and if the purchaser makes an unlawful use of same it is entirely his lookout."

40. Raymond T. Brastow, "Congress and Regulation: The Case of the Pharmaceutical Industry" (Ph.D. diss., University of Washington, 1988).

41. "Harmless Catarrh Powder," *Practical Druggist* 1 (April 1897): 42.

42. Adams, *The Great American Fraud,* 178.

43. "Editorial Notes," *Midland Druggist* (1903): 714.

44. Martin I. Wilbert and Murray Galt Motter, *Digest of Laws and Regulations in Force in the United States Relating to the Possession, Use, Sale, and Manufacture of Poisons and Habit-Forming Drugs* (Washington, D.C.: USPHS, 1912).

45. Adams, *The Great American Fraud,* 42–44.

46. Bureau of Chemistry hearing 144 "Nathan Tucker's Asthma Specific" (September 4, 1908), BC; Monthly Narcotic Returns, "Nathan Tucker Laboratory, Mt. Gilead, Ohio," Bureau of Narcotics, RG 170, National Archives.

47. Adams, *The Great American Fraud,* 43.

48. Mallinckrodt Chemical Works of St. Louis to Essanay Film Company, July 1909, Edward Mallinckrodt, Jr., Papers, Western Historical Manuscript Collection, University of Missouri–St. Louis.

Eight   Consumers' Paradise?

1. Although most historians agree on the nature of the transformation, there is a deep division over its consequences. One interpretation suggests that drug prohibition (usually given as the passage of the federal Harrison Narcotic Act in 1914) changed the world of drug users and sellers from a peaceful, happy one to an underground world of fear, hostility, and crime. Almost immediately after the Harrison Act was passed, writings along this line appeared; for example, Aleister Crowley, *Cocaine* (1918; reprint, San Francisco: Level Press, 1973). More current interpretations include Richard Ashley, *Cocaine: Its History, Uses, and Effects* (New York: Warner Books, 1976) and Joel L. Phillips and Ronald W. Wynne, *Cocaine: The Mystique and the Reality* (New York: Avon Books, 1980). The opposite interpretation of the same trends suggests that the implementation of restrictions on the sale of cocaine was a logical and positive result of increased understanding and information about the drug. David Musto made this argument in "Lessons of the First Cocaine Epidemic," *Wall Street Journal* (June 11, 1996): 31.

2. On the development of the illicit drug trade, see Alan A. Block, "European Drug Traffic and Traffickers between the Wars: The Policy of Suppression and Its Consequences," *Journal of Social History* 23 (Winter 1989): 315–37; Alfred McCoy, *The Politics of Heroin* (New York: Harper & Row, 1991).

3. "A Paper on Cocaine by Dr. William J. Schieffelin," *American Druggist* 48 (1906): 177–78; A. Bingham, police commissioner, New York City, to Hon. Nelson W. Aldrich, May 28, 1909, U.S. Delegation to International Opium Commission and Conferences (hereafter USDIOC).

4. T. D. Crothers, *Morphinism and Narcomanias from Other Drugs* (Philadelphia, 1902), 272. What the tremendous disparity in estimates of legitimate/illegitimate consumption also suggests is the extent to which these categories were exceedingly pliable and inexact. Crothers' estimates, for example, seem to be based upon the percentage of cocaine distributed directly to physicians, dentists, or hospitals, which would undoubtedly have been quite small.

5. "Public Waking Up to Cocaine Menace," *New York Times* (August 3, 1908): 5:5. When New York State finally passed laws regulating the prescribing of cocaine by physicians, the *American Druggist* caustically noted that "physicians must learn what pharmacists have long learned, that the convenience of the individual must be sacrificed to the welfare of the community." "A New Cocaine Law," *American Druggist* (1913): 23.

6. Mallinckrodt Chemical Works to Hamilton Wright, St. Louis Mo., October 20, 1909, USDIOC.

7. Alice Hamilton, *Exploring the Dangerous Trades* (Boston: Little, Brown & Co., 1943), 100–103; see also Barbara Sicherman, *Alice Hamilton: A Life in Letters* (Cambridge: Harvard University Press, 1984).

8. Jane Addams, *Twenty Years at Hull House* (reprint, Chicago: University of Illinois Press, 1990), 173.

9. *Independent* 63 (October 3, 1907): 829–30.

10. Of the fifty-five political divisions reviewed by Martin Wilbert in *Public Health Bulletin* 56 (November 1912), forty-eight restricted the sale of cocaine. So concerned were state legislatures with cocaine that even its close substitutes were tightly regulated. As of 1916, the sale of novocaine was included in anticocaine laws in six states (California, Oregon,

Nebraska, New Jersey, South Dakota, and Utah) and implicitly included in the laws of seven other states. Martin I. Wilbert, memo on novocain, United States Public Health Service (hereafter USPHS), RG 90, file 2123, National Archives.

11. W. J. O'Connor, inspector of police, to Dr. Hamilton Wright, June 22, 1909, US-DIOC.

12. "New York to Have Drastic Cocaine Law," *Pharmaceutical Era* (February 1913): 96. Even after passage of the Harrison Act, the federal government attempted to persuade pharmaceutical manufacturers to confine their production of cocaine to the large crystal variety. In a letter to ten manufacturers, the surgeon general noted that "it has been brought to our attention that the greater part of cocaine hydrochloride produced in this country is of the flaky or small crystal varieties, and that these are the forms in which it is used by the cocaine habitué — it being used almost entirely as a snuff. Note, cocaine hydrochloride also crystallizes in monoclinic prisms, and it has been suggested that its use by habitués might be greatly curtailed if the production was limited to this large crystal variety . . . The bureau is desirous of learning your opinion on this matter, and whether or not you would be willing to limit your output to the large crystal variety." See, for example, Surgeon General to Albany Chemical Company, January 29, 1919, USPHS, RG 90, file 2123, box 205, National Archives. Although it is uncertain whether manufacturers complied with this request, it is clear that the efforts to control cocaine sniffing had the effect of increasing the use of cocaine by hypodermic injection.

13. "Louisiana's New Regulations Governing Sale of Habit Forming Drugs," *Southern Pharmaceutical Journal* (January 1911): 181.

14. "A New Cocaine Ordinance," *Pharmaceutical Era* 34 (November 16, 1905): 455–56, Kremers Reference Files, F. B. Power Pharmaceutical Library, University of Wisconsin–Madison (hereafter KRF).

15. "Cocaine Sellers in Pittsburgh Punished," *American Druggist* 58 (April 24, 1911): 30.

16. "Enforcing the Provisions of the Cocaine and Poison Laws," *Western Pennsylvania Retail Druggist* (hereafter *WPRD*) (March 1911): 14; "A Cocaine Peddler Caught," *WPRD* (April 1911): 8; "Results Following the Recent Cocaine Investigation," *WPRD* (May 1911): 6. The Duquesne druggist's sales violated the first rule of legitimate cocaine sales, as expressed in a *Southern Pharmaceutical Journal* editorial: "Indiscriminate distribution of medicine leads to indiscriminate use, self-medication, and addiction. These vendors do not wait for customers to come to them, but they go to them." "Legislation," *Southern Pharmaceutical Journal* 1 (February 1909): 281.

17. Frederick T. Gordon and E. G. Eberle, "Report of Committee on the Acquirement of Drug Habits," *Proceedings of American Pharmaceutical Association* 51 (1903): 476.

18. Druggists also appeared to have felt rather persecuted by their poor public image problem. The *National Druggist* complained that "the newspapers never appear happier than when they find some pretext for slandering the retail drug trade." "Retail Druggists Make A Brave Fight upon Offenders in Their Ranks," *National Druggist* 40 (July 1910).

19. "Go after Dope Sellers," *Syracuse Herald* (June 21, 1906), KRF.

20. "Board after Cocaine Sellers," *Apothecary* (November 1905): 874.

21. "Crusade against Cocaine," *Midland Druggist* (1903): 925.

22. As Lee Anderson observed, membership in professional organizations was often not particularly strong, even by the mid 1890s. Anderson gives the following participation rates for 1896: Illinois (30% of registered pharmacists), Minnesota (36%), Wisconsin

(47%), New York (16.4%), and Pennsylvania (13.9%). Professional organizations gained strength through the first decade of the twentieth century, however. Although they did not speak for all druggists, these professional organizations claimed what little political power druggists had and helped shape cocaine regulation.

23. "The Responsibilities of Pharmacy," *American Druggist* 43 (September 1903): 235.

24. "Druggists Take the Initiative in Prosecuting Venders of Habit-Forming Drugs," *National Druggist* 40 (May 1910): 203–4.

25. Samuel Hopkins Adams, *The Great American Fraud* (Chicago, 1912), 177–78.

26. In this respect, the National Association of Retail Druggists (NARD) turned to the same approach that physicians had so successfully taken through the American Medical Association.

27. "What Are We Going To Do About It?" *Southern Pharmaceutical Journal* (July 1910): 472.

28. James H. Beal, *An Anti-Narcotic Law* (Detroit, 1903): 1, KRF.

29. A 1907 California law limiting sales of cocaine and opiates to those on prescription of a physician made the California State Board of Pharmacy directly responsible for enforcement. The board was not afraid to exercise its authority against the state's pharmacists. For the fiscal year ending June 30, 1908, the following arrests for violations of narcotics provisions of poison law were made in California: twenty-eight drugstore owners, twenty-four opium den owners, twenty-three drugstore clerks, one drugstore manager, and one messenger boy (from Charles B. Whilden, California State Board of Pharmacy to Hamilton Wright, September 17, 1908, USDIOC).

30. The prosecution of one of the druggists caught in the sweep illustrates the complicated interplay among politics, professional status, and drug control. Emil Graff was arrested for selling cocaine to persons who had no prescription for it. Graff was a prominent Philadelphia druggist who had been a candidate for the Pennsylvania State Pharmaceutical Examining Board shortly before the arrest but had lost to Christopher Koch, who was the man responsible for his arrest! Although the druggists convicted of making illegal sales of morphine received only $75 fines, Graff's cocaine sales earned him a year in prison. It is difficult to determine, in this instance, whether Graff's extreme sentence was a reflection of greater concern over cocaine sales than opiate sales (as happened elsewhere), of political competition, or a combination of both. See "Imprisonment for Selling Cocaine," *Oil, Paint, and Drug Reporter* (June 27, 1910): 76.

31. "Louisville, Ky., Convictions," *Southern Pharmaceutical Journal* 2 (August 1910): 532. A presiding judge in another appeal of the Kentucky law ruled that "the fact as to its legitimate or illegitimate use may be determined by testimony, as in any other issue of fact."

32. "Cocaine Crusade Begins," *Pharmaceutical Era* (December 1, 1904): 560.

33. "The Sale of Cocaine and Cocaine Snuffs," *American Druggist* 42 (March 9, 1903), 124.

34. A. Bingham, police commissioner, New York City, to Hon. Nelson W. Aldrich (May 28, 1909), USDIOC. Bingham's report reappeared in many published articles and reports on the cocaine problem. See, for example, "The Latest Drug Danger," *The World's Work* 18 (August 1909): 11870–71 and also "The Cocaine Habit," *New York Times* (June 20, 1909).

35. *Pharmaceutical Era* (December 21, 1905).

36. How does the consumption of cocaine in New Orleans, a city linked very early to

the growth of popular cocaine use (particularly among its longshoremen), compare with the national totals? The estimates of consumption suggest that in New Orleans it was probably proportionally higher, although it is not clear how much so. In 1909, 5,000 ounces of cocaine represented about 2 percent of the 250,000 ounces that were likely consumed in the United States. The city's population, however, was only 339,075 at the 1910 United States census (or about 0.04% of the U.S. population). Of course, the city's druggists undoubtedly did a substantial business among Louisianans residing outside of the city and among nonresident workers, so these figures can only suggest that New Orleans sold a disproportionate amount of cocaine.

37. Although physicians and druggists had roughly the same access to cocaine, the physicians do not seem to have been responsible for as much of the underground market. As distributors, only a few physicians entered the cocaine business to the extent of a New York City physician who distributed 592 ounces of cocaine in just over three months. Perhaps the most notable exception was reported in 1914 by Ernest Coulter in a letter to Hamilton Wright, in which he observed that a physician in New York City had purchased 6,000 ounces of cocaine in one year! Coulter reported that "this man is now serving a term in Atlanta prison." If this story is true, this would represent the largest single amount of cocaine attributed to one source (all the more remarkable because the legal imports and manufactures of cocaine for 1914 totaled less than 100,000 ounces). Ernest Coulter to Hamilton Wright, September 10, 1914, box 37, USDIOC. A larger role for physicians in the underground market, however, was the sale of prescriptions for cocaine (see below), a market that appears to have become more substantial over time, as more retailers refused sales without a prescription.

38. W. J. O'Connor, inspector of police, to Hamilton Wright, June 22, 1909, USDIOC; St. Clair Adams, New Orleans district attorney to Hamilton Wright, October 17, 1910, US-DIOC.

39. Thomas G. Simonton, "The Increase of the Use of Cocaine among the Laity in Pittsburgh," *Philadelphia Medical Journal* 11 (March 28, 1903): 556–60.

40. "Chicago's Chief Cocaine Seller at Last Defeated," *Druggists Circular* 51 (March 1907): 281.

41. One of the earliest reports of cocaine peddling appeared in a letter from W. Schweckhardt of Dallas to the *American Druggist* in 1894, in which he noted that "at our association meeting recently it was reported that a party was peddling cocaine in the lower quarters of this city." "Cocaine in Texas," *American Druggist* (June 7, 1894): 301–2.

42. "One Effect of the Anti-Cocaine Law," *American Druggist* 52 (February 24, 1908). To a limited extent, the underground market obtained some of its supply through thefts and other illegal diversions from legitimate manufacturers or wholesale firms. The Vice Commission of Chicago illustrated one example of this diversion: "it is practically impossible to ascertain exactly how much cocaine or morphine any particular drugstore buys in spite of the fact that wholesale houses keep a record . . . for instance a clerk in a drugstore at ———— West 22nd street turned in an order for one ounce of cocaine and asked for three ounces, which were given him. The records show he ordered one ounce. This is often done." Vice Commission of Chicago, *The Social Evil in Chicago* (Chicago, 1911), 85. Christopher Koch's 1909–10 investigation of the Philadelphia cocaine network revealed that Benjamin P. Ashmead, U.S. government inspector of drugs at the port of Philadelphia, used his position to supply druggists in the city with cocaine. Employees at the city's three largest

wholesale firms were also involved. One was arrested for having stolen hundreds of ounces of cocaine in one year from his employer, and three others were arrested for selling cocaine to two peddlers. Much of the supply, however, followed legal channels to the retail druggist. In some respects, this early illegitimate market bears some resemblance to the current distribution network of illegal sedatives, tranquilizers, amphetamines, and methadone, where much of the supply comes from product obtained illegally from physicians or druggists. See, for example, Dana E. Hunt, "Drugs and Consensual Crimes: Drug Dealing and Prostitution," in *Drugs and Crime*, ed. Michael Tonry and James Q. Wilson (Chicago: University of Chicago Press, 1990), 159–202.

43. Chicago *Record-Herald* (December 19, 1911).

44. See Alan A. Block and William J. Chambliss, "Organizing the Cocaine Trade," in *Organizing Crime* (New York: Elsevier, 1981), 43–60. Fred Williams suggested a somewhat more centralized source of supply in San Francisco, with five important distributors of cocaine ("Foxy" Maloney, "Pine Street Pete," "Hard Luck Pat," "Turk Street Paul," and "Sammie the Moor") in San Francisco by 1920, below whom operated countless street-level dealers of the drug. Fred V. Williams, *The Hop-Heads: Personal Experiences among the Users of 'Dope' in the San Francisco Underworld* (San Francisco, 1920).

45. One of the most notable exceptions was the Swann anticocaine ordinance passed by the city of Baltimore which made the possession of cocaine a crime. Although city officials felt the ordinance to be effective, their experiment was not duplicated in many other places, including the state of Maryland, whose legislature refused to extend the Swann Law to the remainder of the state.

46. Regulations against registered druggists, on the other hand, were much tighter. The explanation for this discrepancy was that, as noted above, state pharmacy boards had the authority to regulate the practice of pharmacy. Consequently, pharmacy boards could, and did, put limits on the *possession* of cocaine by druggists.

47. C. H. Theobald to J. S. Abbott, Texas Food and Drug Commissioner, August 18, 1913, Bureau of Chemistry.

48. "The Cocaine Evil," *The Outlook* (February 8, 1913): 292; "Cocaine Law Construed," *New York Times* (September 27, 1908): 20:4.

49. "Much Cocaine Found in Raid," *New York Times* (September 10, 1911) 8:1.

50. Thomas A. McQuaide to Hamilton Wright, June 29, 1909, USDIOC.

51. Harris Dickson to Hamilton Wright, December 7, 1909, USDIOC.

52. "Aaron Martin Sold 470 Ounces of Cocaine in Nine Months," *New Orleans Item*, USDIOC.

53. Vice Commission of Chicago, *The Social Evil in Chicago*, 243–44.

54. Ibid., 243.

55. Williams, *The Hop-Heads*, chap. 25.

56. Other adulterants included boric acid and magnesium sulfate (Epsom salts).

57. Williams, *The Hop-Heads*.

58. In 1909, the state of Kentucky and federal authorities, seeking to break up the trade in cocaine between New Albany, Indiana, and Louisville (situated across the Ohio River), solicited cocaine from Charles Crescilius, a New Albany druggist. They received two shipments of cocaine powder, each packaged in falsely labeled boxes and containing acetanilide mixed with 18.14 percent and 19.64 percent cocaine. Kentucky, whose state cocaine laws were tightly enforced, found itself battling the free supply of cocaine from the druggists of

New Albany, where regulations prohibiting the "promiscuous" sale of cocaine went largely unenforced. Bureau of Chemistry, interstate seizure files 2838-b and 2839-b "Cocaine," Food and Drug Administration. Louisville authorities directed most of their criticism at the New Albany public prosecutor, Walter Bullett, who consistently refused to prosecute local druggists for cocaine selling. See *Report of the Kentucky Board of Pharmacy* (1910), US-DIOC. At the request of the Kentucky Board of Pharmacy, agents of the Bureau of Chemistry obtained evidence to prosecute Crescilius for interstate shipment of misbranded and adulterated cocaine.

59. New Orleans *Item* (July 16, 1900 and September 19, 1900); two observations may be made concerning Simon's sales of cocaine. First, the amount of cocaine Simon sold for 5¢ was probably about a half-grain, which would have cost the druggist about a penny. Second, a comparison of New Orleans in 1900 and Musto's New York in 1908 indicates that cocaine was about twice as expensive in 1908 as it had been in 1900. The comparison suggests that although the retail price of cocaine in the underground market had begun to rise before 1908, it continued to do so throughout the pre–Harrison Act era.

60. The *Literary Digest* seems to have been quoting a writer from the *New York Sun,* who also suggested that the coke fiend spent about $4 to $5 per day by 1914. Of course, newspaper reporting standards were notoriously low. Although the *New York Sun* claimed that the use of cocaine required "more money than any other drug addiction exacts," the *New York World* suggested that "Cocain and its allied intoxicants appear to be about the cheapest things in the market."

61. E. R Waterhouse, "Cocaine Debauchery," *Eclectic Medical Journal* 56 (1896): 464–65.

62. Block and Chambliss, "Organizing the Cocaine Trade."

63. Police Commissioner Bingham to Nelson W. Aldrich, May 28, 1909, USDIOC.

64. The first druggist convicted under the city's 1907 anticocaine ordinance was Charles Hitsch, a Chinatown druggist. In November 1907, Hitsch was sentenced to six months of imprisonment in the state penitentiary, after his third conviction. "New York Cocaine Seller Imprisoned," *American Druggist* 51 (November 1907): 749.

65. The responses to Wright are in the "New York" file of the Wright Papers. See also Hamilton Wright, "General Statistics" and "New York Notes" in USDIOC.

66. Adams, *The Great American Fraud,* 41–42.

67. Block and Chambliss, "Organizing the Cocaine Trade, 57."

68. Frank L. McGuire to Hamilton Wright, August 4, 1908, USDIOC.

69. Simonton, "The Increase of the Use of Cocaine among the Laity of Pittsburgh," 556.

70. "Special Report," August 26, 1914, vol. 87, folder 4, Charles Merriam Papers, University of Chicago Special Collections, Joseph Regenstein Library, Chicago, Ill.

71. Harris Dickson to Hamilton Wright, USDIOC.

Conclusion

1. Drug prohibition is frequently defended on moral grounds; several years ago James Q. Wilson observed that the costs associated with drug use "are to a large degree moral . . . the heavy consumption of certain drugs is destructive of human character." James Q. Wil-

son, "Drugs and Crime," in *Crime and Justice: A Review of Research,* vol. 13 (Chicago: University of Chicago Press, 1990), 523.

2. Ethan A. Nadelmann, "Drug Prohibition in the United States: Costs, Consequences, and Alternatives," *Science* 245 (1989): 939–47.

3. Alfred R. Lindesmith, *Opiate Addiction* (Bloomington, Ind.: Principia Press, 1947).

4. Others have taken a similar position. Kildare Clarke concluded of medicalizing currently illicit forms of drug use, "The scorn of drug use and abuse would be removed, to be replaced with the same level of care given to all other medical problems." See Kildare Clarke, "Legalization of Drugs and Beyond Legalization," in *Searching for Alternatives: Drug-Control Policy in the United States,* ed. Melvyn B. Krauss and Edward P. Lazear (Stanford: Hoover Institution Press, 1991), 424–34.

5. Christopher Wren, "Study Poses a Medical Challenge to Disparity in Cocaine Sentences," *New York Times* (November 20, 1996): A1, A11.

6. Lester Grinspoon and James B. Bakalar, "Marihuana as Medicine: A Plea for Reconsideration," *JAMA* 273 (1995): 1875–76.

7. Avram Goldstein and Harold Kalant, "Drug Policy: Striking the Right Balance," *Science* 249 (1990): 1513–22. For another articulation of harm reduction, see Don C. Des Jarlais, "Harm Reduction: A Framework for Incorporating Science into Drug Policy," *American Journal of Public Health* 85 (1995): 10–12, in which he observes that "the harm reduction perspective emphasizes the need to base policy on research rather than on stereotypes of (legal and illegal) drug users." Legalization proposals share with harm reduction proposals some reliance on medical authority. See, for example, Richard B. Karel, "A Model Legalization Proposal," in *The Drug Legalization Debate,* ed. James A. Inciardi (Newbury Park, Calif.: Sage Publications, 1991), 80–102.

8. J. B. Mattison, "Cocaine Dosage and Cocaine Addiction," *Peoria Medical Monthly* 7 (1886–87): 572–73.

9. Lewis H. Adler, "The Status of the Hydrochlorate of Cocaine in Minor Surgery, as Based upon the Experiences of Philadelphia Physicians," *Therapeutic Gazette* 7 (1891): 518.

10. The "consolidation of professional authority" is the subject of *The Social Transformation of American Medicine* by Paul Starr (New York: Basic Books, 1982). Starr's work provides the context within which the attitude toward cocaine in the medical/pharmaceutical professions may be understood. On the subject of reform more generally, these conclusions hearken back to the descriptions of reform outlined by Gabriel Kolko in *The Triumph of Conservatism* (New York: Free Press, 1963) and given further elaboration by James Weinstein in *The Corporate Ideal in the Liberal State, 1900–1918* (Boston: Beacon Press, 1968).

11. There is a large, and growing, body of historical literature which aims to locate the agency of various subjects of social control efforts. The earliest of these dealt with working-class women, as in the case of Christine Stansell, *City of Women: Sex and Class in New York, 1790–1860* (New York: Alfred A. Knopf, 1986) and Kathy Peiss, *Cheap Amusements: Working Women and Leisure in Turn-of-the-Century New York* (Philadelphia: Temple University Press, 1986) as well as working-class blacks in Robin D. G. Kelley, "The Black Poor and the Politics of Opposition in a New South City, 1929–1970," in *The "Underclass" Debate: Views from History,* ed. Michael Katz (Princeton: Princeton University Press, 1993), 293–333. Other important areas of historical work include studies of prostitution, especially Timothy Gilfoyle, *City of Eros: New York City, Prostitution, and the Commercialization*

of Sex, 1790–1920 (New York, Norton, 1992), and gay subcultures, especially George Chauncey, *Gay New York: Gender, Urban Culture, and the Making of the Gay Male World, 1890–1940* (New York: Basic Books, 1994). The more recent of these, especially Kelley and Chauncey, owe a great deal to the work of James C. Scott, *Domination and the Arts of Resistance: Hidden Transcripts* (New Haven: Yale University Press, 1990), which argues that marginalized groups challenge power by asserting their own form of political culture — one expressed through everyday activities.

SOURCES

PRIMARY SOURCES

A Note on Manuscript Sources

The most important primary sources employed in this work were those that detailed the actions of cocaine manufacturers and distributors. In the course of my preliminary investigations, I was impressed with the potential of sources related to distribution to reveal broader patterns of cocaine *consumption* in the United States. Moreover, as a legal enterprise (albeit a highly competitive and secretive one), cocaine manufacturing and selling were chronicled more extensively than a comparable illicit enterprise.

I believed at the outset that the records of pharmaceutical and chemical firms would provide the most valuable information. Comprehensive documentation of cocaine manufacturing from this period, however, is difficult to obtain. It is worth remembering that even Hamilton Wright, in the service of the U.S. delegation to the International Opium Conference in 1908 and 1909, was repeatedly refused even the most basic information regarding cocaine production among large manufacturers. Problems of access still exist, although some major pharmaceutical firms are in the process of making their early records available to historical researchers. One hopes that this trend will continue and help give the American pharmaceutical industry its deserved prominence in the history of American business and manufacturing.

One significant focus of research involved the activities of Parke, Davis & Company, the leading American promoter and producer of cocaine. Documenting the activities of Parke, Davis suggests both the limitations and the potential of company records. The most interesting materials are in the Parke, Davis & Company Collection, part of the Burton Historical Collections of the Detroit Public Library. These materials, deposited at the library during one of the company's relocations, contain a remarkable collection of company records from the 1860s through the 1950s. At the heart of the collection are the records of various departments from the 1890s through the 1910s, including pills manufacture, private formulas, fluid extracts, hypodermic tablets, and specialties. The records provide fascinating details of the day-to-day operations of the company, including experimentation and production details. Unfortunately, the majority of the collection is not cataloged, with the documents exactly in the condition that the company delivered them.

A second source of information regarding Parke, Davis and the pharmaceutical industry in general is in the Kremers Reference Files of the American Institute of the History of Pharmacy (AIHP). The files, located on the campus of the University of Wisconsin–Madison, are a unique and eclectic collection begun before World War II by Edward Kremers, the second head of the university's pharmacy program. Reorganized after the war and recently moved to a new storage facility, the files are readily accessible and organized by categories such as pharmaceutical manufacturing, retail pharmacy, pharmacy education, materia medica, and biographical information. For a more detailed description, see Gregory J. Higby and Elaine C. Stroud, "Pharmaco-Historical Resources in Madison, Wisconsin: Kremers Reference Files," *Pharmacy in History* 30 (1988): 157–62. Among the materials useful for this study were items regarding the activities and publications of Parke, Davis researchers Albert Lyons and Henry Rusby (including personal correspondence from the latter) and a small but fascinating collection of materials from the Parke, Davis plant superintendent.

The single most valuable source of information regarding the operations of Parke, Davis was the F. E. Stewart Papers (1866–1938). The Stewart papers are part of the AIHP Collection located at the Wisconsin Historical Society in Madison (mss. 606). The heart of the collection is the professional correspondence between Dr. Francis Edward Stewart, consulting physician to Parke, Davis for much of the 1880s, and the man primarily responsible (George S. Davis) for founding the scientific department of the company. Stewart's long career eventually took him to H. K. Mulford & Company, where he founded its scientific department as well. What makes these papers so valuable is the extensive correspondence between Stewart and Davis regarding Stewart's ongoing role in developing and marketing new remedies in the 1880s, including cocaine.

The collections of the AIHP include a large number of company catalogs and price lists. Equally substantial are the collections of the Lloyd Library and Museum in Cincinnati. The Lloyd Library is the product of a collection of pharmacy-related publications and materials begun by the Lloyd brothers, whose pharmaceutical firm was based in Cincinnati. The library collection "Drug Price Lists and Circulars, 1870–1970" contains many useful items, including the only copies I found of the Mariani publication, *The Coca Leaf.* In addition, the records of the Mallinckrodt Chemical Works, which include a part of the Edward Mallinckrodt Papers and are housed at the University of Missouri–St. Louis, provide enormously helpful insight into the chemical manufacturing enterprise.

As complicated as it is to document the activities of an ethical drug maker such as Parke, Davis, the operations of patent medicine manufacturers are even more obscure. Indeed, most of what we know regarding these firms comes from the unrepresentative few who survived to the present (such as Coca-Cola) and from surviving advertisements, packages, and circulars. One pathway into understanding the operations of patent medicine makers, however, was suggested to me by the work of James Harvey Young, who has spent decades documenting the dark side of the patent medicine business. The records of the U.S. Food and Drug Administration (Rockville, Maryland) include case files of proceedings against violators of the Pure Food and Drug Act, undertaken by the bureaucratic predecessor of the FDA, the Bureau of Chemistry. These records are organized by case number and include substantial files on catarrh and asthma cures, coca wines, soft drinks, and even individual druggists whom the bureau attempted to prosecute under federal food and drug laws.

The activities of retail druggists are fairly well documented; many historical societies, for example, contain the business records of one or more pharmacies. By their nature, such records are difficult to employ systematically. In this work, I used records of individual drugstores deposited at the AIHP, the Detroit Public Library, and the Michigan Historical Collection of the Bentley Historical Library in Ann Arbor.

Finally, two other important sources should be noted here, although each has been used previously by other historians. The first comprises the collections of the History of Medicine Division of the National Library of Medicine in Bethesda, Maryland. In addition to a remarkable collection of rare published materials, the library houses the Lawrence Kolb Manuscript Collection. Although Kolb, one of the nation's leading authorities on drug use and drug addiction, concentrated his efforts on opiate addiction, there are also useful materials pertaining to cocaine.

The second source is the collections housed in the National Archives, including the U.S. Public Health Service Records (record group 90) and the Records of the U.S. Delegations to the International Opium Commission and Conferences, 1909–1913 (record group 43). The latter set of records includes a remarkable volume of correspondence between Hamilton Wright, who was a member of the delegation, and representatives of drug manufacturers, wholesalers, and law enforcement. Much of the correspondence is the result of two surveys conducted by Wright. The first, in 1908, dealt largely with opium consumption. The second, in 1909, focused on trends and problems associated with cocaine consumption. The responses provide, at the very least, an important snapshot of official opinion regarding the "cocaine problem" near the peak of consumption.

Journals

The large number of medical and pharmaceutical journals published during the time period covered by this study provided ample material with which to gauge professional sentiment regarding the use and distribution of cocaine. I have listed only those journals whose contents I attempted to review systematically, including the dates covered. In all cases, the journals were part of collections of either the Falk Library of the Health Sciences at the University of Pittsburgh or the F. B. Power Library at the School of Pharmacy, University of Wisconsin–Madison.

American Druggist and Pharmaceutical Record (1884–1920)
American Journal of Pharmacy (1915)
Apothecary (1904–6)
Boston Medical and Surgical Journal (1884–1920)
Bulletin of Pharmacy (1890–1910)
Canadian Pharmaceutical Journal (1905–12)
Druggists' Circular (1907–10)
Journal of the American Medical Association (1884–1920)
Journal of the American Pharmaceutical Association (1884–1920)
Medical Age (1885)
Medical News (1884–1905)
Merck's Report (1905)
Meyer Brothers Druggist (1899)
Midland Druggist (1902–3)
National Druggist (1884–1918)
New Orleans Medical and Surgical Journal (1880–85)
New York Medical Journal (1884–1920)
Oil, Paint, and Drug Reporter (1880–1920)
Pharmaceutical Era (1888–1920)
Pittsburgh Druggist (1885–94)

Practical Druggist (1896–97)
Quarterly Journal of Inebriety (1888–1910)
Southern Pharmaceutical Journal (1908–14)
Therapeutic Gazette (1880–86)
Western Pennsylvania Retail Druggist (1910–18)

Contemporary Publications

Adams, Samuel Hopkins. *The Great American Fraud*. Chicago: American Medical Association Press, 1912.

Bartholow, Roberts. *A Practical Treatise on Materia Medica and Therapeutics,* 5th ed. New York: D. Appleton & Co., 1884.

——— . *A Practical Treatise on Materia Medica and Therapeutics,* 10th ed. New York: D. Appleton & Co., 1900.

Beal, James H. *An Anti-Narcotic Law*. Detroit: William M. Warren, 1903.

Beard, George M. *American Nervousness: Its Causes and Consequences*. New York: G. P. Putnam's Sons, 1881.

——— . *A Practical Treatise on Nervous Exhaustion (Neurasthenia): Its Symptoms, Nature, Sequences, Treatment*. New York: E. B. Treat, 1880.

Bishop, Ernest S. *The Narcotic Drug Problem*. New York: Macmillan Co., 1920.

Bunting, Charles A. *Hope for the Victims of Alcohol, Opium, Morphine, Cocaine, and Other Vices*. New York: Christian Home Building, 1888.

Coca. Philadelphia: William R. Warner & Co., 1885.

Crothers, T.D. *The Drug Habits and Their Treatment*. Chicago: G. P. Engelhard & Co., 1902.

——— . *Inebriety*. Cincinnati: Harvey Publishing Co., 1911.

——— . *Morphinism and Narcomanias from Other Drugs: Their Etiology, Treatment, and Medicolegal Relations*. Philadelphia: W. B. Saunders & Co., 1902. Reprint, New York: Arno Press, 1981.

Dai, Bingham. *Opium Addiction in Chicago*. Reprint, Montclair, N.J.: Patterson Smith, 1970.

Dercum, Francis X., ed. *A Text-Book on Nervous Diseases*. Philadelphia: Lea Brothers & Co., 1895.

Flowers, Montaville, and H. R. Bonner. *The Menace of Morphine, Heroin and Cocaine*. Pasadena, Calif.: Narcotic Education Association, 1923.

Hare, Hobart Amory. *A Text-Book of Practical Therapeutics,* 5th ed. Philadelphia: Lea Brothers & Co., 1895.

Kolb, Lawrence, and A. G. Du Mez. *The Prevalence and Trend of Drug Addiction in the United States and Factors Influencing It*. Washington, D.C.: GPO, 1924.

Lewin, Louis. *Phantastica: Narcotic and Stimulating Drugs, Their Use and Abuse*. Munich: P. H. A. Wirth, 1924. Reprint, New York: E. P. Dutton, 1964.

Lloyd, John Uri. *Origin and History of All the Pharmacopeial Vegetable Drugs*. Cincinnati: Caxton Press, 1929.

——— . *A Treatise on Coca (Erythroxylon Coca): The "Divine Plant of the Incas."* Cincinnati: Lloyd Brothers, 1913.

Maier, Hans W. *Der Kokainismus*. Translated by Oriana Josseau Kalant. Toronto: Addiction Research Foundation, 1987.

Mariani, Angelo. *Coca Erythroxylon (Vin Mariani): Its Uses in the Treatment of Disease,* 4th ed. New York: Mariani & Co., 1886.

——— . *Coca and Its Therapeutic Applications,* 2d ed. New York: J. N. Jaros, 1892.

Martindale, William. *Coca and Cocaine: Their History, Medical and Economic Uses, and Medicinal Preparations,* 3d ed. London: H. K. Lewis, 1894.

Mortimer, W. Golden. *Peru: History of Coca, "The Divine Plant" of the Incas.* New York: J. H. Vail & Co., 1901.

Parke, Davis & Company. *Coca Erythroxylon and Its Derivatives.* Detroit: George S. Davis, [1885?].

——— . *The Pharmacology of the Newer Materia Medica.* Detroit: George S. Davis, 1892.

Rusby, Henry H. *Jungle Memories.* New York: Whittlesey House, 1933.

Rusby, Henry H., A. Richard Bliss, and Charles W. Ballard. *The Properties and Uses of Drugs.* Philadelphia: P. Blakiston's Son & Co., 1930.

Sainsbury, Harrington. *Drugs and the Drug Habit.* New York: E. P. Dutton, 1909.

Searle, William S. *A New Form of Nervous Disease (Together with an Essay on Erythroxylon Coca).* New York: Fords, Howard & Hulbert, 1881.

Street, John Phillips. *The Composition of Certain Patent Proprietary Medicines.* Chicago: American Medical Association, 1917.

Terry, Charles E., and Mildred Pellens. *The Opium Problem.* New York: Bureau of Social Hygiene, 1928.

——— . *Preliminary Report in Studies of the Use of Narcotics under the Provisions of Federal Law in Six Communities.* New York: Bureau of Social Hygiene, 1924.

Towns, Charles B. *Drug and Alcohol Sickness.* New York: M. M. Barbour Co., 1932.

U.S. Department of the Treasury. *Traffic in Narcotic Drugs: Report of the Special Committee of Investigation Appointed March 25, 1918, by the Secretary of the Treasury.* Washington, D.C.: GPO, 1919.

Vice Commission of Chicago. *The Social Evil in Chicago: A Study of Existing Conditions with Recommendations.* Chicago: Gunthorp-Warren Printing Co., 1911.

Wilbert, Martin I. *The Number and Kind of Drug Addicts.* Washington, D.C., U.S. Public Health Service, 1915.

Wilbert, Martin I., and Murray Galt Motter. *Digest of Laws and Regulations in Force in the United States Relating to the Possession, Use, Sale, and Manufacture of Poisons and Habit-Forming Drugs.* Washington, D.C.: U.S. Public Health Service, 1912.

Williams, Fred V. *The Hop-Heads: Personal Experiences among the Users of "Dope" in the San Francisco Underworld.* San Francisco: Walter N. Brunt, 1920.

Woods, Arthur. *Dangerous Drugs: The World Fight against Illicit Traffic in Narcotics.* New Haven: Yale University Press, 1931.

Woods, H. C. *Therapeutics: Its Principles and Practice,* 8th ed. Philadelphia: J. B. Lippincott Co., 1891.

SECONDARY SOURCES

Many published works have contributed to the development of this study. The notes to each chapter identify and discuss these secondary sources in some detail. This note on sources summarizes the most important of these, to guide those interested in pursuing further inquiry in specific subject areas.

Current historical scholarship in the area of illicit drugs and their legal control owes a great deal to three landmark works: David F. Musto, *The American Disease* (New York: Oxford University Press, 1973; expanded ed., 1987), still the most comprehensive survey of American drug control; Virginia Berridge and Griffith Edwards, *Opium and the People: Opiate Use in Nineteenth-Century England* (New Haven: Yale University, 1987); and David T. Courtwright, *Dark Paradise: Opiate Addiction in America before 1940* (Cambridge: Harvard University Press, 1982). Their work has been the inspiration for more recent studies, including Jill Jonnes, *Hep-Cats, Narcs, and Pipe Dreams: A History of America's Romance with Illegal Drugs* (New York: Scribner, 1996); Marek Kohn, *Dope Girls: The Birth of the British Drug Underground* (London: Lawrence & Wishart, 1992); and Jim Baumohl, "The 'Dope Fiend's Paradise' Revisited: Notes from Research in Progress on Drug Law Enforcement in San Francisco, 1875–1915," *Surveyor* 24 (June 1992): 3–12.

The legal and medical use of cocaine has been the subject of less historical attention than that of opiates. The most interesting of the early works on cocaine is Robert Byck, ed., *Cocaine Papers by Sigmund Freud* (New York: Stonehill, 1975), an outstanding compilation of primary sources. Other valuable edited works include: George Andrews and David Solomon, *The Coca Leaf and Cocaine Papers* (New York: Harcourt Brace Jovanovich, 1975); Lise Anglin, *Cocaine: A Selection of Annotated Papers from 1880 to 1894 Concerning Health Effects* (Toronto: Addiction Research Foundation, 1985); and Joel L. Phillips, *A Cocaine Bibliography* (Rockville, Md.: National Institute on Drug Abuse, 1974). Lester Grinspoon and James B. Bakalar, *Cocaine: A Drug and Its Social Evolution* (New York: Basic Books, 1976) offers a very useful account of the early history of coca. The most recent work, Steven B. Karch, *A Brief History of Cocaine* (Boca Raton, Fla.: CRC Press, 1998), details the international cocaine trade before World War II.

The drug industry, in ethical and patent medicine variations, still has not received as much attention from historians as it deserves. The historical literature is growing, however, and includes a number of very important works. On the ethical industry and pharmaceutical science, see Louis Galambos with Jane Eliot Sewell, *Networks of Innovation: Vaccine Development at Merck, Sharp and Dohme, and Mulford, 1895–1995* (New York: Cambridge University Press, 1995); Jonathan Liebenau, *Medical Science and Medical Industry: The Formation of the American Pharmaceutical Industry* (Baltimore: Johns Hopkins University Press, 1987); John Parascandola, *The Development of American Pharmacology: John J. Abel and the Shaping of a Discipline* (Baltimore: Johns Hopkins University Press, 1992); John P. Swann, *Academic Scientists and the Pharmaceutical Industry: Cooperative Research in Twentieth-Century America* (Baltimore: Johns Hopkins University Press, 1988). On the patent medicine trade, a lifetime of work is ably covered in James Harvey Young, *American Health Quackery: Collected Essays by James Harvey Young* (Princeton: Princeton University Press, 1992). For a better understanding of the relationship among medical practice, the drug business, and pharmacological knowledge, the following (very different) works are valuable: Harry M. Marks, *The Progress of Experiment: Science and Therapeutic Reform in the U.S., 1900–1990* (New York: Cambridge University Press, 1997); Paul Starr, *The Social Transformation of American Medicine* (New York: Basic Books, 1982); and John Harley Warner, *The Therapeutic Perspective: Medical Practice, Knowledge, and Identity in America, 1820–1885* (Cambridge: Harvard University Press, 1986).

The historical literature on other forms of illicit trades not only provides the context for the cocaine business but also suggests ways in which the underground drug trade might be better understood. Important general works in this area include: Alan A. Block and William J. Chambliss, *Organizing Crime* (New York: Elsevier, 1981); John C. Burnham, *Bad Habits: Drinking, Smoking, Taking Drugs, Gambling, Sexual Misbehavior, and Swearing in American History* (New York: New York University Press, 1993); Mark Haller, "Organized Crime in Urban Society: Chicago in the Twentieth Century," *Journal of Social History* 5 (Winter 1971–72): 210–34; and James A. Inciardi and Charles E. Faupel, eds., *History and Crime: Implications for Criminal Justice Policy* (London: Sage Publications, 1980). Recent monographs on various "underground" trades and cultures are too numerous to mention here, but two that have been most helpful are: George Chauncey, *Gay New York: Gender, Urban Culture, and the Making of the Gay Male World, 1890–1940* (New York: Basic Books, 1994) and Timothy J. Gilfoyle, *City of Eros: New York City, Prostitution, and the Commercialization of Sex, 1790–1920* (New York: Norton, 1992).

Finally, there is an immense contemporary literature on illicit drug distribution and drug control policy to which historians should pay greater attention. This is particularly true of the many ethnographic investigations of the drug trade, including: Patricia Adler, *Wheeling and Dealing: An Ethnography of an Upper-Level Drug Dealing and Smuggling Community* (New York: Columbia University Press, 1985); Phillipe Bourgois, *In Search of Respect: Selling Crack in El Barrio* (New York: Cambridge University Press, 1996); and Terry Williams, *Cocaine Kids* (Reading, Mass.: Addison-Wesley, 1989). Other studies of drug selling include: Peter Reuter, Robert MacCoun, and Patrick Murphy, *Money from Crime: A Study of the Economics of Drug Dealing in Washington, D.C.* (Santa Monica, Calif.: RAND Corporation, 1990) and Vincenzo Ruggerio and Nigel South, *Eurodrugs: Drug Use, Markets and Trafficking in Europe* (London: UCL Press, 1995). An indispensable review of policy issues, with much historical insight, is Franklin E. Zimring and Gordon Hawkins, *The Search for Rational Drug Control* (New York: Cambridge University Press, 1992).

INDEX

Library of Congress Cataloging-in-Publication Data

Spillane, Joseph.
   Cocaine : from medical marvel to modern menace in the
United States, 1884–1920 / Joseph F. Spillane.
     p. cm. — (Studies in industry and society : 18)
   Includes bibliographical references and index.
   ISBN 0-8018-6230-2 (alk. paper)
    1. Cocaine habit—United States—History. 2. Cocaine—
United States—History. 3. Cocaine industry—United States
—History. 4. Narcotics, Control of—United States—History.
I. Title. II. Series.
HV5825.S597 2000
362.29'8'0973—dc21   99-32725
                                          CIP